Mental Health and Nursing Care of Individuals with Cancer and Their Families

Mental Health and Nursing Care of Individuals with Cancer and Their Families

Editor

Margaret Fitch

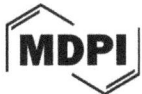

Basel • Beijing • Wuhan • Barcelona • Belgrade • Novi Sad • Cluj • Manchester

Editor
Margaret Fitch
Bloomberg Faculty of Nursing
University of Toronto
Toronto
Canada

Editorial Office
MDPI
St. Alban-Anlage 66
4052 Basel, Switzerland

This is a reprint of articles from the Special Issue published online in the open access journal *Healthcare* (ISSN 2227-9032) (available at: www.mdpi.com/journal/healthcare/special_issues/cancer_nursing).

For citation purposes, cite each article independently as indicated on the article page online and as indicated below:

Lastname, A.A.; Lastname, B.B. Article Title. *Journal Name* **Year**, *Volume Number*, Page Range.

ISBN 978-3-0365-9667-9 (Hbk)
ISBN 978-3-0365-9666-2 (PDF)
doi.org/10.3390/books978-3-0365-9666-2

© 2023 by the authors. Articles in this book are Open Access and distributed under the Creative Commons Attribution (CC BY) license. The book as a whole is distributed by MDPI under the terms and conditions of the Creative Commons Attribution-NonCommercial-NoDerivs (CC BY-NC-ND) license.

Contents

About the Editor vii

Preface ix

Keren Dopelt, Noam Asna, Mazal Amoyal and Osnat Bashkin
Nurses and Physicians' Perceptions Regarding the Role of Oncology Clinical Nurse Specialists in an Exploratory Qualitative Study
Reprinted from: *Healthcare* **2023**, *11*, 1831, doi:10.3390/healthcare11131831 1

Ching-Hui Cheng, Shu-Yuan Liang, Ling Lin, Tzu-Ting Chang, Tsae-Jyy Wang and Ying Lin
Caregiving Self-Efficacy of the Caregivers of Family Members with Oral Cancer—A Descriptive Study
Reprinted from: *Healthcare* **2023**, *11*, 762, doi:10.3390/healthcare11050762 14

Hiroko Komatsu and Yasuhiro Komatsu
The Role of Nurse on the Treatment Decision Support for Older People with Cancer: A Systematic Review
Reprinted from: *Healthcare* **2023**, *11*, 546, doi:10.3390/healthcare11040546 23

Sukhuma Klankaew, Suthisa Temthup, Kittikorn Nilmanat and Margaret I. Fitch
The Effect of a Nurse-Led Family Involvement Program on Anxiety and Depression in Patients with Advanced-Stage Hepatocellular Carcinoma
Reprinted from: *Healthcare* **2023**, *11*, 460, doi:10.3390/healthcare11040460 40

Meinir Krishnasamy, Heidi Hassan, Carol Jewell, Irene Moravski and Tennille Lewin
Perspectives on Emotional Care: A Qualitative Study with Cancer Patients, Carers, and Health Professionals
Reprinted from: *Healthcare* **2023**, *11*, 452, doi:10.3390/healthcare11040452 53

Chia-Chi Hsiao, Suh-Ing Hsieh, Chen-Yi Kao and Tsui-Ping Chu
Development of a Scale of Nurses' Competency in Anticipatory Grief Counseling for Caregivers of Patients with Terminal Cancer
Reprinted from: *Healthcare* **2023**, *11*, 264, doi:10.3390/healthcare11020264 65

Ellen Karine Grov and Siri Ytrehus
Do You Feel Safe at Home? A Qualitative Study among Home-Dwelling Older Adults with Advanced Incurable Cancer
Reprinted from: *Healthcare* **2022**, *10*, 2384, doi:10.3390/healthcare10122384 79

Laura-Anne Aitken and Syeda Zakia Hossan
The Psychological Distress and Quality of Life of Breast Cancer Survivors in Sydney, Australia
Reprinted from: *Healthcare* **2022**, *10*, 2017, doi:10.3390/healthcare10102017 92

Yuri Nakai, Yusuke Nitta and Reiko Hashimoto
Intervention of Coordination by Liaison Nurse Where Ward Staff Struggled to Establish a Therapeutic Relationship with a Patient Because of Failure to Recognize Delirium: A Case Study
Reprinted from: *Healthcare* **2022**, *10*, 1335, doi:10.3390/healthcare10071335 107

Normarie Torres-Blasco, Rosario Costas-Muñiz, Lianel Rosario, Laura Porter, Keishliany Suárez and Cristina Peña-Vargas et al.
Psychosocial Intervention Cultural Adaptation for Latinx Patients and Caregivers Coping with Advanced Cancer
Reprinted from: *Healthcare* **2022**, *10*, 1243, doi:10.3390/healthcare10071243 116

About the Editor

Margaret Fitch

Dr Margaret Fitch has been an oncology nurse, educator, and researcher for more than 25 years. She has contributed many publications and presentations at national and international conferences. She is currently a Professor (Adjunct) in the Faculty of Nursing and the School of Graduate Studies at the University of Toronto.

Preface

As individuals face a cancer diagnosis and are treated for this disease, they will face changes, challenges, and life-changing consequences. Emotional distress can emerge to a greater or lesser degree and have a significant impact on the quality of life. Nurses have an important role in identifying emotional distress and mental health challenges.

The articles in this collection offer insights and enhanced understanding of mental health and nursing care of individuals and their families facing the emotional distress of confronting a life-threatening illness.

I appreciate the authors who have contributed to this Special Issue and provided their perspectives on the topics from different parts of the world.

Margaret Fitch
Editor

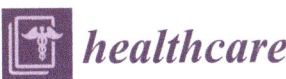

Article

Nurses and Physicians' Perceptions Regarding the Role of Oncology Clinical Nurse Specialists in an Exploratory Qualitative Study

Keren Dopelt [1,2,*,†], Noam Asna [3,†], Mazal Amoyal [4] and Osnat Bashkin [1]

1. Department of Public Health, Ashkelon Academic College, Ashkelon 78211, Israel; osnatba@edu.aac.ac.il
2. School of Public Health, Faculty of Health Sciences, Ben Gurion University of the Negev, Beer Sheva 84105, Israel
3. Oncology Institute, Shaare Zedek Medical Center, Jerusalem 91031, Israel; asnaoffice@yahoo.com
4. Palliative Care Unit, Barzilai Medical Center, Ashkelon 78306, Israel; mazalam@bmc.gov.il
* Correspondence: dopelt@bgu.ac.il; Tel.: +972-8-6789-503
† These authors contributed equally in this work.

Abstract: The purpose of the study was to examine the attitudes of nursing and medical teams about the role of oncology clinical nurse specialists in the healthcare system in Israel, where, unlike many countries in the world, such a role has not yet been developed or professionally defined. We conducted 24 interviews with physicians and nurses between August and October 2021. The interviews were transcribed and analyzed using a thematic analysis method. The Consolidated Criteria for Reporting Qualitative Research checklist was used to report the study. Five main themes emerged from the interviews: (1) contribution to the healthcare system, (2) contribution to the patient, (3) drawing professional boundaries, (4) additional responsibilities and authority for oncology clinical nurse specialists, and (5) the field's readiness for a new position of oncology clinical nurse specialists. The findings provide evidence about the need to develop the role of clinical nurse specialists in the oncology field due to its potential benefits for nurses, physicians, patients, family members, and the healthcare system. At the same time, an in-depth exploration of the boundaries of the role and its implementation, in full cooperation with the oncologists and relevant professional unions, is needed to prevent unnecessary conflicts in the oncology field. Professional development training programs in nursing must create a platform for open dialogue between key stakeholders, nurses, and physicians, in order to help all involved parties, place the benefits to the patients above any personal or status considerations.

Keywords: oncology; nursing; clinical nurse specialists; cancer patients; expanding nurses' authority; professionalization; policy; education

1. Introduction

Israel has approximately 200,000 cancer patients, with some 29,000 new cases annually [1]. The oncology field involves complex clinical treatments and deals with complicated psychosocial issues associated with patients and their family members [2]. In recent decades, countries throughout the world have developed medical support positions, such as clinical nurse specialists, as a strategy to meet the healthcare system's challenges. Studies show that clinical nurse specialists can provide the necessary medical care in situations meeting the position's definitional framework and, in a manner, offering the optimal response to patients' needs [3–5]. In the United States, there are about 300,000 clinical nurse specialists, and in the United Kingdom, about 3300, whereas in Israel, there are only 358 clinical nurse specialists working in the fields of supportive care (102), geriatrics (80), diabetes (32), surgery (30), premature infants (28), pain (8), rehabilitation (4), and policy and administration (74) [6].

There are barriers and disagreements regarding the definition, authority, and recognition of this role in Israel's healthcare system, which make it difficult to expand it to other clinical areas [7]. Oncology nursing is a challenging and evolving profession that requires regular updating about both the medical aspects of the disease and the mental and social factors related to its diagnosis and treatment [8]. The oncology clinical nurse specialist can improve patients' health outcomes and quality of life indicators [9] and thereby increase patients' satisfaction with the treatment and involvement in disease management [10,11]. Moreover, integrating clinical nurse specialists leads to decreased rates of hospitalization, mortality, and complications [12].

A recent study in Israel examined the experiences of 39 clinical nurse specialists in supportive care. The nurses reported dissatisfaction with the work environment and with how their role was recognized and implemented by hospital physicians and managers. In addition, the limited authority they were granted did not correspond to the description of the role [13]. These findings are consistent with the results of a previous study conducted in Canada, which found barriers to the implementation and assimilation of clinical nurse specialists, including the lack of a model to guide the implementation of the role, lack of an agreed-upon description of the role and responsibilities; and lack of ongoing support and mentorship [14].

Despite the positive evidence of the inherent benefits of oncology clinical nurse specialists, there is disagreement about the role's definition and necessity. A study that examined the perceptions of this role in the field of oncology found that definitions of the position were unclear. While physicians and managers perceived the role of an oncology clinical nurse specialist as "helping" medical practitioners in managing their workloads, the oncology clinical nurse specialists themselves perceived their role as promoting holistic, patient-centered care and proactively meeting the unique oncology patients' needs [11]. Conflicts concerning the boundaries of the role, lack of resources and organizational and systemic support, and physicians' fear that clinical nurse specialists will replace them limit the potential of the role and reduce its essential contribution to quality care in oncology [11].

The growing number of cancer patients and their multiple needs, the shortage of oncologists, and the rapid changes in the clinical, organizational, and technological environment in the field of oncology highlight the need to update the clinical and managerial skills of oncology nurses. The literature shows that oncology clinical nurse specialists offer many advantages. However, in contrast to many countries around the world (the United States, Canada, the United Kingdom, Japan, Brazil, and others), in Israel, the position of an oncology clinical nurse specialist has not yet been established. Implementation of this role in the healthcare system in Israel depends to a large extent on a characterization of the position, understanding its benefits for the healthcare system and the patients, and an in-depth understanding of the barriers to its implementation that must be taken into account already at the planning stage. The purpose of the present study is to examine the potential contribution of oncology clinical nurse specialists as seen through the eyes of medical and nursing professionals.

2. Methods

We conducted an exploratory qualitative study using semi-structured interviews. The study was approved by the Ashkelon Academic College Ethics Committee (Approval No. 20-2020). The Consolidated Criteria for Reporting Qualitative Research (COREQ) checklist was used to report the study.

2.1. Population and Procedure

Semi-structured in-depth interviews were conducted between August and October 2021, after informed consent was obtained from twenty-four healthcare professionals from various medical centers in all geographical parts of Israel, using purposeful sampling. Purposeful sampling is a non-random sampling technique that uses specific criteria or purposes to select a sample [15]. The aim is to collect in-depth information from the right respondents. The inclusion criteria: oncology doctors or nurses, doctors or nurses in the position of decision-makers, or clinical nurse specialists. We continued the interviews until theoretical saturation was reached. To recruit interviewees, we contacted people working in the field of oncology and invited them to take part in the study. We asked each participant to provide the name of a colleague who would be willing to participate in the research. Among the twenty-four interviewees, six were physicians and eighteen nurses. Seven interviewees were males, and seventeen were females. All interviews were conducted over the telephone due to COVID-19 social distancing restrictions and were audiotaped and transcribed verbatim in Hebrew. It was emphasized to the interviewees that their details would remain confidential, no findings would be published under their name, and they did not have to answer all the questions, or they could stop the interview. The interviewer was a Clinical Psychology graduate student, trained in qualitative research methods and supervised by KD and OB. There was no relationship between the interviewer and the participants. The interviews lasted between 30 and 50 min.

2.2. Study Tool

The in-depth interview guide was developed in collaboration with oncology staff members and drew on our literature reviews. The interview guide was validated using the content validation method by two oncology nurses and two physicians to ensure that the questions were relevant to the study goals. The guide was pilot tested with one oncology nurse to ensure a smooth interview flow and verify comprehension of the questions. Information collected during the interviews included perceptions toward the role of nurses in cancer care and the need to develop oncology clinical nurse specialists training (Appendix A).

2.3. Data Analysis

The interviews were transcribed accurately by a professional and analyzed using a thematic analysis method based on grounded theory [16] in the ATLAS.ti v.8 software (Berlin, Germany). The Grounded Theory method uses both an inductive and a deductive approach to theory development. Our analysis included incorporating deductive themes arising from the research topics and based on a literature review of quality in cancer care and cancer survivors' needs, together with inductive themes that emerged from the data [17]. The interpretive analysis was done close to the interviews in several stages: (1) the interviews were read at least once by KD and OB to gain in-depth knowledge of the data. (2) KD and OB identified ideas, categories, and themes related to the study's objectives. (3) central themes were redefined to include encoded quotes and examples based on re-reading the transcripts. Relevant passages were marked and allocated to one of the content themes. The themes and quotes were examined iteratively by all authors and documented in English at the final stage. The description of the findings was accompanied by citations from the interviewees and thus provided continuous evidence for matching the interpretation and the interviewees' unique voices.

3. Results

3.1. Participants' Characteristics

Participants' characteristics and codification are available in Table 1.

Table 1. Characteristics of the interviewees (P = Physician, N = Nurse).

Code	Gender	Role
P1	Male	Hospital Oncologist, Head of the Oncology department
P2	Male	Community family physician, Member of the National Secretariat of the Israel Medical Association (IMA)
P3	Female	Hospital Oncologist
P4	Male	Hospital and Community Oncologist, Head of the Oncology department

Table 1. Cont.

Code	Gender	Role
P5	Male	Hospital and Community Oncologists
P6	Male	Public Health physician, Board member of the Organization of State Employee Physicians, IMA
N1	Female	Senior nurse, working at the Department of professional development in Nursing Management, the Ministry of Health
N2	Female	Hospital Oncology nurse
N3	Female	Community Oncology nurse
N4	Female	Community Palliative nurse
N5	Female	Community Palliative nurse
N6	Female	Community Palliative and Oncology nurse
N7	Female	Hospital Oncology nurse
N8	Female	Hospital Oncology nurse, Board member of the Association for Oncology Nursing
N9	Female	Hospital Palliative nurse, also working at the Nursing Management, the Ministry of Health
N10	Female	Hospital clinical nurse specialist
N11	Male	Hospital Palliative nurse
N12	Female	Hospital Palliative and radiotherapy nurse
N13	Female	Senior Nurse, Head of the ambulatory division in a hospital, including Oncology and Hematology clinics
N14	Female	Hospital Palliative nurse
N15	Female	Senior Nurse, Department of professional development in the Nursing Management, the Ministry of Health
N16	Female	Hospital Palliative nurse, breast cancer specialist
N17	Female	Hospital Palliative nurse
N18	Female	Head of the hospital nursing oncology division

3.2. Main Themes

Five main themes emerged from the interviews: (1) contribution to the healthcare system, (2) contribution to the patient, (3) drawing professional boundaries, (4) additional responsibilities and authority for oncology clinical nurse specialists, (5) the field's readiness for a new position of oncology clinical nurse specialists. A conceptual map of the main categories is presented in Figure 1.

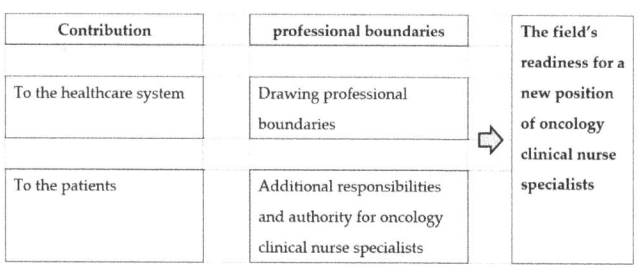

Figure 1. A conceptual map of the main categories.

The themes, with quotes that illustrate each, are presented in Tables 2–6.

Table 2. Theme 1—Contribution to the healthcare system.

Quotes
"Knowing how to get a person settled back at home, for example, can reduce hospitalizations. When a patient goes home with instructions and is in contact with a clinical nurse specialist, this will reduce visits to the emergency room and hospitalizations and contributes to the wellbeing of the patient and the family." (N16)
"If there are nurses who know how to respond and do physical examinations and observe the patients' problems before the physician arrives, that would help. Many times, a physician just reviews the tests and does not have time to physically see the patients and talk to them." (N4)
"We have a clinical nurse specialist in surgery for the emergency room. She does more than half of the work, so the doctor is freed up to do surgery. She makes diagnoses. She sends for imaging. The patient is not delayed and doesn't have to wait for the physician to come from the operating room." (N14)
"This could certainly provide a solution to the distress and pressure we live with. I don't think there is competition here. There is enough load on the system." (P4)
"You need a clinical specialist nurse in practically every field. Certainly, in oncology, the patient needs the emotional support aspect. Being with them, the support, is very, very important. Also, a nurse who knows the patient well can give personalized care, tailored to the patient." (N10)
"Nurses complement physicians' work—and I emphasize: complement not replace. They do not need to replace a physician's work—they need to complement a physician's work. The medical profession must be maintained. I come from within the system and understand the constraints of the system. Therefore, I allow myself to say that I do not agree with the [response to the] constraints of the system, that if there is a shortage of physicians, nurses are brought in." (P6)
"The goal of the nursing administration is to promote the nursing profession, not the system. Despite our evidence, as physicians, that she improves patient care." (P2)

Table 3. Theme 2—Contribution to the patient.

Quotes
"Today, oncology is looking towards the community. People live with metastatic disease for many years, and they live in their community. A person can receive chemotherapy or biological therapy with pills in the community, without going to an inpatient department at a hospital or a radiation institute. Also, the population is older, people live longer, and they have underlying diseases as well as cancer. That's why the treatments are more and more often given in the community. And this will continue." (N8)
"You can reduce referrals to the emergency room. All patients run to the emergency room, but the emergency room is a very difficult experience for the patient. It exposes them to infections, and they wait for many hours. If someone in the community will go to the patient and take care of things that a nurse can do at the patient's home, it will be great for everyone." (N3)
"No one sees the patient as a whole, all the various aspects related to dealing with his medical condition. And I think that nursing, specifically, is a field that really keeps an overall view of the patient." (N5)
"Many patients in the community fall through the cracks, they are neither here nor there. There are oncology patients in advanced stages, but not yet in hospice or terminal. They need follow-up. A clinical nurse specialist in oncology can provide the solution." (N3)
"The nurse frees me from the secondary things. This does not free me from seeing the patient, from providing treatment and instructions. But it improves service to the patient." (P5)

Table 4. Theme 3—Drawing professional boundaries.

Quotes
"What will this contribute to oncology? They [CNS] will learn how to alleviate pain and symptoms. What can a nurse contribute more than a clinical nurse specialist in palliative care does? Beyond that, someone could only prescribe chemotherapy, and I don't think anyone [a nurse] would want to take that on herself." (N9)
"Specifically for oncology? I think there is such a shortage of nurses, that this seems to me like a luxury. As it is, there are not enough nurses, in my opinion." (N16)
"It will hurt the quality of treatment. It cuts into the professional authority that until now has been given to physicians. It also hurts the physician's status and standing. The physicians feel that their authority is being undermined. Instead of making the effort to find, train, and employ enough physicians, they bring in personnel of lower quality to do things that are proper medical functions. The result of all this diminishes the quality of medical services. Maybe it's in exchange for increased availability, because there are more nurses. But it's definitely a reduction of quality." (P6)
"The medical profession has only two unique aspects: making a diagnosis and providing treatment. Only a physician can do those things. Whether there is a need for a mid-level practitioner in oncology is a question you should ask oncologists. I think there is. Should that mid-level practitioner be a nurse? In my opinion, no. They should talk to us, the physicians, about this, and it should be done in a way that is cooperative and not adversarial ... In many professions, this is not a real need in the system. If there is a real need in the system and we need personnel who are not physicians, we need to create assistant physicians, then we will have an additional profession and will not take the best nursing minds away from nursing and towards medicine, when we already have a shortage in nursing." (P2)
"There can't be any confusion between professions. Nurses have enough to do. I am not sure they should also be given options that require a broad understanding of the patient. In this case, openness is based on a misrepresentation of the problem of job standards. The problem of standards is that an informed decision is made by the people who control the flow of money. You don't have to abolish the professional criteria to cover the money that is going to other places." (P1)

Table 5. Theme 4—Additional responsibilities and authority for oncology clinical nurse specialists.

Quotes
"The difference between a nurse in an oncology ward and a clinical nurse specialist is their authority and in-depth learning. [They can do] things that an ordinary nurse doesn't have the authority to do: prescribe medications, give referrals for tests, make decisions regarding treatment. At the same time, they have excellent psychosocial skills. [They know] how to communicate with families and people in complicated situations, [to deal] with ethical dilemmas, to support a person at the end of life, and to manage a decision-making process in cooperation with the patient and the family." (N8)
"The added value is that she can provide a sense of balance to patients. She will outline the treatment. Today, she receives instructions from a physician. But if she has the whole range of knowledge about the treatments, the indications, she will have room to take independent action. If we have a clinical nurse specialist in oncology, she will need, for example, to have the ability to respond and make a medical decision about starting a new medication." (P1)

Table 6. Theme 5—Conflicts of oncology clinical nurse specialists' professional status.

Quotes
"I don't know if the field is ready. How many of the other teams, such as physicians or paramedical teams understand what this role is, what it includes, how to cooperate with that role? Here, I think it might be a little more problematic." (N2).
"I think that even now there is not full implementation of the responsibilities that already exist. There is a lot of complexity around it. I don't know if I would be involved in expanding the list of responsibilities, but I would be involved in seeing that what is already on the list is carried out." (N16)
"There are physicians who accept it, and there are physicians who have a hard time with it—mostly physicians in the community. Physicians in the hospital love the [clinical nurse] specialists because, for them, this is another significant help in treating the patient." (N18)
"I think physicians also understand that this is important. The future is going in that direction. If the United States already had this thirty years ago, accepting nurse specialists [working] independently is very common there, so there is no reason why it couldn't happen in Israel. In my case, some raised their eyebrows and said, 'Who are you, as a nurse, to tell me what to do?'" (N10)
"Only if you are weak, then you are afraid of the rise of the nurse. The nurse will not take my place. But she is my right hand." (P5)

Theme 1—Contribution to the healthcare system.

Nurses and physicians described multiple benefits of oncology clinical nurse specialists to the healthcare system:

1. Reducing and alleviating the burden on physicians;
2. Improving service and treatment for patients;
3. Reducing hospitalizations;
4. Creating a professional role at an intermediate level that can help patients;
5. Providing a perspective that advances the profession of nursing.

However, some physicians argue that the solution to the workforce problem is to add physicians and not to transfer responsibilities to nurses.

Theme 2—Contribution to the patient.

In terms of contribution to the patient, interviewees mentioned a response that is holistic and available and reduces bureaucracy and waiting time. It is particularly important to integrate the role of clinical nurse specialists into community healthcare settings and to improve services and support for convalescents. The nurse will maintain continuity in the transition between the hospital and the community. This can reduce the need for hospitalization to receive further treatment and alleviate the burden on physicians so that most treatment for convalescents will occur in community settings.

Theme 3—Drawing professional boundaries.

Clinical nurse specialists in various fields expressed concern about the Ministry of Health's unwillingness to grant real responsibility to clinical nurse specialists. They also described dilemmas regarding nurses' willingness to take on the responsibility of managing treatments or administering medications.

According to the physicians' perception:

1. In practice, nurses know how to recommend the proper pain relief medications, but do not have the authority to prescribe them. A physician must make referrals for tests and approve the administration of any medications because, ultimately, the physician is responsible for the patient;
2. Creating a role for clinical nurse specialists unnecessarily "wastes" the nursing workforce. A nurse does not need to be a physician's assistant. For this purpose, paramedics, for example, can be trained;

3. Politically, the process of creating a new role with expanded responsibilities must be coordinated with the physicians' unions so that it will have their support and recognition and not be perceived as "eroding" the physicians' role. There is a fear that physicians' status will change as a result, or that there will be discomfort regarding the quality of nursing personnel in the healthcare system;
4. In terms of administrative hierarchy, there is a question as to whether clinical nurse specialists will be subordinate to the director of the nursing department or to the head physician of the relevant department since the clinical nurse specialist has authority similar to that of a physician.

Theme 4—Additional responsibilities and authority for oncology clinical nurse specialists.

Nurses suggested expanding the responsibilities of oncology clinical nurse specialists to include:

1. Prescribing pain-relieving medications;
2. Giving referrals for tests (i.e., blood tests, imaging);
3. Interpreting test results for patients;
4. Giving referrals to other professionals (nutritionists, pharmacists, etc.);
5. Participating in making therapeutic decisions;
6. Managing the treatment according to structured protocols;
7. Assisting the patient during the transition back into the community;
8. Calling the patient/family with updates.

Physicians suggested that the position of OCNS should include the following:

1. Providing a holistic response to patients, especially in terms of follow-up and transition back into the community
2. Providing long-term follow-up for patients after the intensive treatment; this would be a unique added value of the position of administering pain-relieving medications.

Theme 5—Conflicts of oncology clinical nurse specialists' professional status.

Oncology nurses raised concerns about how physicians would accept oncology clinical nurse specialists. Clinical nurse specialists in other fields mentioned the gaps between the job definition compared to their actual responsibilities and the current situation in the field. The main gap pertained to prescriptions for medications given by nurse specialists, which the Pharmacists Ordinance does not recognize. So, despite their professional knowledge and experience in giving prescriptions, their authority is not recognized in practice. Another issue is that the nurses' responsibilities are not being implemented, making it difficult to grant them more extensive responsibilities. Clinical nurse specialists described the challenges in the implementation process and gaining recognition of their role by the physicians. All nurses mentioned the importance of recognition of this role by physicians.

Physicians referred to the importance of implementing and defining the role in order to promote cooperation in the workplace so that more physicians will recognize clinical specialists as having the knowledge and authority to give advice and as people who can offer teaching and training.

4. Discussion

The current study aimed to examine the perceptions of nursing and medical teams about the role of oncology clinical nurse specialists. The findings reveal a complex picture regarding the OCNS role and the need for expanding nurses' authority. The delegation of authority from physicians to nurses represents one of the most important elements in the professionalization process of nursing [18] and expanding nurses' authority is a significant contributor to professional autonomy [19]. Various studies describe positive attitudes of physicians and nurses toward expanding nurses' authority in several areas based on their belief that this will improve the quality of care [20–22].

The oncology nurses, some of the clinical nurse specialists, the nurses from the Ministry of Health nursing management, and the oncology physicians were unanimous about the need for oncology clinical nurse specialists' role and about the ability of the nurses to serve as case managers. Nurses related that they see the development of an oncology clinical nurse specialist as an opportunity for professional development, especially in community healthcare settings. From an oncologist's perspective, oncology clinical nurse specialists provide a reliable, professional workforce that can relieve their burden and improve the quality of service to the patient.

Our findings are consistent with other studies conducted around the world indicating the importance of the oncology clinical nurse specialists in several aspects: improving cancer diagnosis and treatment services [23]; preventing the need for hospitalization and emergency services [23,24]; reducing hospitalizations [25]; issuing faster and more accurate therapeutic prescriptions; providing a reliable, accessible, and available source of information [26]; and providing psychosocial support for patients and their family members [27,28].

According to interviewees, the oncology clinical nurse specialist role can offer the added value of comprehensive treatment because currently, no single healthcare professional performs the function of providing overall management of the treatment. Similarly, Griffiths [29] reported that oncology clinical nurse specialists view the treatment of cancer patients from a holistic perspective. Brooten [30] finds an economic rationale for expanding the authority of oncology clinical nurse specialists because they provide high-quality care while potentially reducing healthcare's high costs, given that they earn significantly lower wages than physicians.

In the United Kingdom, clinical nurse specialists provide care once performed by physicians (prescribing medications, making diagnoses), thereby reducing the burden on physicians [31], shortening waiting times for receiving oncology services, and making treatment accessible to patients who live in peripheral areas [32]. Since 2010, the Australian government has been operating rural oncology clinics managed by oncology clinical nurse specialists to bridge gaps in access to oncology services between big cities and remote areas [9,33]. Therefore, a training and implementation model for clinical nurse specialists in oncology will empower nurses, benefit patients, reduce healthcare costs, and relieve the burden on oncology physicians, especially in peripheral areas suffering from a lack of physicians.

Despite all the inherent advantages and potential of the oncology clinical nurse specialists, some of the clinical specialist nurses and physicians from professional organizations thought that such a position is not necessary, and that even if extra assistance is needed, it can be provided by physician assistants (for example, paramedics who will undergo appropriate training) and not necessarily by a clinical nurse specialist nurse. Reasons given for this approach included: possible erosion of physicians' status; physicians not recognizing the role and broad responsibilities of clinical nurse specialists; objections to compromising and accepting fewer professional personnel rather than increasing the number of physicians; and ambiguity regarding the role and the need for a clear and precise definition its responsibilities. Oncology nurses also raised concerns about a lack of recognition of the role on the part of the doctors. The scientific literature frequently mentions topics such as tension with other professionals, intruding on the responsibilities of other professionals in a way that harms teamwork, and ambiguity of the role of clinical specialists working in a multidisciplinary team [34]. Other studies have found that the main challenges in implementing this role are a poor understanding of it among decision-makers, lack of clarity about the role, lack of support from management, and misunderstanding of it among the medical staff [35–37]. Additionally, previous studies have documented condemnations of the role and criticisms of inappropriate and wasteful use of nursing personnel [27]. All these reasons mentioned in the interviews in the current study and in previous studies indicate that interviewees and researchers in the field agree that it is necessary to define clear responsibilities for the clinical nurse specialists and the maximum limits of the role's authority [27,38].

Given the global shortage of medical and nursing staff, the World Health Organization (WHO) stated in the Munich Declaration [39] that healthcare systems must develop new roles for nurses working in hospitals and in the community. The interviewees in the current study said they think that the new role is crucial for community healthcare. Many cancer patients are treated in community healthcare settings, and cancer survivors need treatment and follow-up care in the community. Continuity between treatment in hospitals and community healthcare clinics has a considerable effect on oncology patients. Studies show that such continuity is linked to high patient satisfaction, improved quality of life and mental health indicators [40,41], improved responsiveness to treatment, and better therapist-patient communication [42]. In contrast, lack of treatment continuity was found to be related to increases in the use of unnecessary medical services [43], hospitalizations, and visits to emergency medical facilities [42].

Cancer requires complex treatment, the use of different sections of the healthcare system, and multiple caregivers. Patients and their families frequently report a lack of information concerning treatments, professionals, ways to communicate with healthcare providers, and above all, how to navigate the healthcare system [44]. Oncology clinical nurse specialists can fill this vacuum and play a key role in facilitating cancer patients' encounters with the system. Support for this role was found both in research in the field of oncology and in studies that examined managing chronic care by nurses [45–48].

Study Limitations

The sample is limited but is considered reasonable for exploratory studies using qualitative research methodology [49]. We made efforts to include a wide range of stakeholders related to the research topic from various settings and regions in Israel in order to obtain responses from a broad and diverse swath of the healthcare system in Israel. Moreover, the interviews were transcribed from Hebrew, the native language of Israel. This may have increased the chances for variations in the interpretation of our data. We made all efforts to ensure methodological rigor and validity of the translations from Hebrew to English by using a standardized codebook, meeting frequently, sharing and comparing our results, and performing a pilot analysis. Throughout the study, we conducted an internal quality audit during our meetings, adapted from Tong et al. [50], to determine whether the data were collected, analyzed, and reported consistently according to the study protocol.

5. Conclusions

Multidisciplinary, coordinated, and holistic treatment may respond to the psychosocial and clinical issues facing the oncology field. The findings of this study provide evidence about the need to develop a new role of oncology clinical nurse specialists in Israel due to its potential benefits for nurses, physicians, patients, family members, and the healthcare system as a whole. At the same time, the conclusions drawn from the study reveal a complex challenge. An in-depth exploration of the boundaries of the role and its implementation, in full cooperation with the oncologists and relevant professional unions, is needed to prevent unnecessary conflicts in the oncology field. Professional development training programs in the nursing field must create a platform for dialogue between management and key stakeholders of nursing and medical departments in order to help all involved parties place the benefits to the patients first, and above any personal or status considerations. The role of oncology clinical nurse specialists can potentially impact the quality of care, prevent hospitalizations, alleviate the pressure and burden on physicians, and reduce costs for the healthcare system. In addition, we recommend extending the responsibilities of oncology nurses to those that exist in various countries around the world (e.g., Germany, Australia, the United States, etc.) and formally designating them as treatment managers. Additionally, we recommend that more nurses be available in the community to provide support, companionship, and follow-up to cancer survivors. Based on these findings, we recommend further research examining cancer patients' attitudes toward this suggested new role in oncology nursing in Israel.

Author Contributions: Conceptualization: K.D., O.B., N.A. and M.A.; Methods design: K.D. and O.B.; Managing data curation: K.D. and O.B.; Analysis and interpretation: K.D., O.B. and N.A.; Writing—original draft: K.D. and N.A.; Review and editing final draft: O.B., K.D., N.A. and M.A. All authors have read and agreed to the published version of the manuscript.

Funding: This work was supported by the National Institute for Health Services Research and Health Policy, Israel (Grant number 2020/120).

Institutional Review Board Statement: The study was conducted according to the guidelines of the Declaration of Helsinki and approved by the Ethics Committee of Ashkelon Academic College (Approval # 20-2020).

Informed Consent Statement: Written informed consent was obtained from all participants in the study. No personal information of participants is published in the article.

Data Availability Statement: The data that support the findings of this study are available from the corresponding author.

Conflicts of Interest: The authors declare no conflict of interest.

Appendix A Interview Guide

1. Tell me a little about yourself, your current role, and any previous noteworthy roles you performed.
2. What do you know about the role of a clinical nurse specialist in Israel and worldwide? How about developing clinical expertise among nurses, arguments for and against?
3. What do you think is the contribution of a clinical specialist nurse to patients and the healthcare system?
4. In Israel today, there are clinical specialists in nursing in only six fields. Do you think the role of a clinical specialist nurse in oncology is required in Israel? In the hospital? In the community? In both? What do you think its added value is?
5. In your opinion, what should the functions and authority of a hospital oncological nurse include?
6. In your opinion, what should the functions and authority of a community oncological nurse include?
7. In your opinion, does the development of clinical specialists erode the authority and status of doctors?
8. From your experience—how was the role of clinical specialist nurse received by both the nurses and the doctors? Did you feel the resistances and barriers that you had to remove? Can you give examples?
9. Would you like to add anything?

References

1. Israel National Cancer Registry. *Cancer Incidence Table*; Israeli Ministry of Health: Jerusalem, Israel, 2021.
2. Dopelt, K.; Bashkin, O.; Asna, N.; Davidovitch, N. Health locus of control in cancer patient and oncologist decision-making: An exploratory qualitative study. *PLoS ONE* **2022**, *17*, e0263086. [CrossRef] [PubMed]
3. Alessy, S.A.; Lüchtenborg, M.; Rawlinson, J.; Baker, M.; Davies, E.A. Being assigned a clinical nurse specialist is associated with better experiences of cancer care: English population-based study using the linked National Cancer Patient Experience Survey and Cancer Registration Dataset. *Eur. J. Cancer Care* **2021**, *30*, e13490. [CrossRef] [PubMed]
4. Balsdon, H.; Wilkinson, S. A trust-wide review of clinical nurse specialists' productivity. *Nurs. Manag.* **2014**, *21*, 33–37. [CrossRef] [PubMed]
5. Birrell, F.; Leung, H.Y. The Scottish prostate cryotherapy service-the role of the clinical nurse specialist. *Br. J. Nurs.* **2019**, *28*, S12–S16. [CrossRef]
6. Khaklai, Z. *Personnel in the Health Professions 2020*; The Information Department, Israeli Ministry of Health: Jerusalem, Israel, 2021.
7. Aaron, E.M.; Andrews, C.S. Integration of advanced practice providers into the Israeli healthcare system. *Isr. J. Health Policy Res.* **2016**, *5*, 7. [CrossRef]
8. Kadmon, I.; Halag, H.; Dinur, I.; Katz, A.; Zohar, H.; Damari, M.; Cohen, M.; Levin, E.; Kislev, L. Perceptions of Israeli women with breast cancer regarding the role of the Breast Care Nurse throughout all stages of treatment: A multi-center study. *Eur. J. Oncol. Nurs.* **2015**, *19*, 38–43. [CrossRef]

9. Challinor, J.M.; Alqudimat, M.R.; Teixeira, T.O.A.; Oldenmenger, W.H. Oncology nursing workforce: Challenges, solutions, and future strategies. *Lancet Oncol.* **2020**, *21*, e564–e574. [CrossRef]
10. Andregård, A.C.; Jangland, E. The tortuous journey of introducing the nurse practitioner as a new member of the healthcare team: A meta-synthesis. *Scand. J. Caring Sci.* **2015**, *29*, 3–14. [CrossRef]
11. Stahlke-Wall, S.; Rawson, K. The Nurse Practitioner Role in Oncology: Advancing Patient Care. *Oncol. Nurs. Forum.* **2016**, *43*, 489–496. [CrossRef]
12. Newhouse, R.P.; Stanik-Hutt, J.; White, K.M.; Johantgen, M.; Bass, E.B.; Zangaro, G.; Wilson, R.F.; Fountain, L.; Steinwachs, D.M.; Heindel, L.; et al. Advanced practice nurse outcomes 1990–2008: A systematic review. *Nurs. Econ.* **2011**, *29*, 230–251.
13. Haron, Y.; Romem, A.; Greenberger, C. The role and function of the palliative care nurse practitioner in Israel. *Int. J. Palliat. Nurs.* **2019**, *25*, 186–192. [CrossRef] [PubMed]
14. Sangster-Gormley, E.; Martin-Misener, R.; Downe-Wamboldt, B.; Dicenso, A. Factors affecting nurse practitioner role implementation in Canadian practice settings: An integrative review. *J. Adv. Nurs.* **2011**, *67*, 1178–1190. [CrossRef] [PubMed]
15. Campbell, S.; Greenwood, M.; Prior, S.; Shearer, T.; Walkem, K.; Young, S.; Bywaters, D.; Walker, K. Purposive sampling: Complex or simple? Research case examples. *J. Res. Nurs.* **2020**, *25*, 652–661. [CrossRef]
16. Chun Tie, Y.; Birks, M.; Francis, K. Grounded theory research: A design framework for novice researchers. *SAGE Open Med.* **2019**, *7*, 2050312118822927. [CrossRef] [PubMed]
17. Shkedi, A. *Words That Try to Touch: Qualitative Research-Theory and Application*; Ramot: Tel-Aviv, Israel, 2003. (In Hebrew)
18. Henderson, V. The concept of nursing. *J. Adv. Nurs.* **2006**, *53*, 21–34. [CrossRef] [PubMed]
19. Jones, K. Developing a prescribing role for acute care nurses. *Nurs. Manag.* **2009**, *16*, 24–28. [CrossRef]
20. De Baetselier, E.; Dilles, T.; Batalha, L.M.; Dijkstra, N.E.; Fernandes, M.I.; Filov, I.; Friedrichs, J.; Grondahl, V.A.; Heczkova, J.; Helgesen, A.K.; et al. Perspectives of nurses' role in interprofessional pharmaceutical care across 14 European countries: A qualitative study in pharmacists, physicians and nurses. *PLoS ONE* **2021**, *16*, e0251982. [CrossRef]
21. Ling, D.L.; Hu, J.; Zhong, M.Y.; Li, W.T.; Yu, H.J. Attitudes and beliefs towards implementation of nurse prescribing among general nurses and nurse specialists in China: A cross-sectional survey study. *Nurs. Open* **2021**, *8*, 2760–2772. [CrossRef]
22. Pursio, K.; Kankkunen, P.; Sanner-Stiehr, E.; Kvist, T. Professional autonomy in nursing: An integrative review. *J. Nurs. Manag.* **2021**, *29*, 1565–1577. [CrossRef]
23. National Cancer Action Team. *Excellence in Cancer Care: The Contribution of the Clinical Nurse Specialist*; NCAT: London, UK, 2010.
24. Corner, J. The role of nurse-led care in cancer management. *Lancet Oncol.* **2003**, *4*, 631–636. [CrossRef]
25. Baxter, J.; Leary, A. Productivity gains by specialist nurses. *Nurs. Times* **2011**, *107*, 15–17. [PubMed]
26. Borland, R.; Glackin, M.; Jordan, J. How does involvement of a hospice nurse specialist impact on the experience on informal caring in palliative care? Perspectives of middle-aged partners bereaved through cancer. *Eur. J. Cancer Care* **2014**, *23*, 701–711. [CrossRef] [PubMed]
27. Kerr, H.; Donovan, M.; McSorley, O. Evaluation of the role of the clinical Nurse Specialist in cancer care: An integrative literature review. *Eur. J. Cancer Care* **2021**, *30*, e13415. [CrossRef]
28. Morgan, B.; Tarbi, E. The Role of the Advanced Practice Nurse in Geriatric Oncology Care. *Semin. Oncol. Nurs.* **2016**, *32*, 33–43. [CrossRef]
29. Griffiths, P.; Simon, M.; Richardson, A.; Corner, J. Is a larger specialist nurse workforce in cancer care associated with better patient experience? Cross-sectional study. *J. Health Serv. Res. Policy* **2013**, *18*, 39–46. [CrossRef]
30. Brooten, D.; Youngblut, J.M.; Kutcher, J.; Bobo, C. Quality and the nursing workforce: APNs, patient outcomes and health care costs. *Nurs. Outlook* **2004**, *52*, 45–52. [CrossRef] [PubMed]
31. Ream, E.; Wilson-Barnett, J.; Faithfull, S.; Fincham, L.; Khoo, V.; Richardson, A. Working patterns and perceived contribution of prostate cancer clinical nurse specialists: A mixed method investigation. *Int. J. Nurs. Stud.* **2009**, *46*, 1345–1354. [CrossRef] [PubMed]
32. Farrell, C.; Molassiotis, A.; Beaver, K.; Heaven, C. Exploring the scope of oncology specialist nurses' practice in the UK. *Eur. J. Oncol. Nurs.* **2011**, *15*, 160–166. [CrossRef]
33. Crawford-Williams, F.; Goodwin, B.; March, S.; Ireland, M.J.; Hyde, M.K.; Chambers, S.K.; Aitken, J.F.; Dunn, J. Cancer care in regional Australia from the health professional's perspective. *Support. Care Cancer* **2018**, *26*, 3507–3515. [CrossRef]
34. Cook, O.; McIntyre, M.; Recoche, K.; Lee, S. "Our nurse is the glue for our team"—Multidisciplinary team members' experiences and perceptions of the gynaecological oncology specialist nurse role. *Eur. J. Oncol. Nurs.* **2019**, *41*, 7–15. [CrossRef]
35. Bryant-Lukosius, D.; Green, E.; Fitch, M.; Macartney, G.; Robb-Blenderman, L.; McFarlane, S.; Bosompra, K.; DiCenso, A.; Matthews, S.; Milne, H. A survey of oncology advanced practice nurses in Ontario: Profile and predictors of job satisfaction. *Nurs. Leadersh.* **2007**, *20*, 50–68. [CrossRef]
36. Delamaire, M.; Lafortune, G. *Nurses in Advanced Roles: A Description and Evaluation of Experiences in 12 Developed Countries*, OECD Health Working Papers, No. 54; OECD Publishing: Paris, France, 2010. [CrossRef]
37. DiCenso, A.; Martin-Misener, R.; Bryant-Lukosius, D.; Bourgeault, I.; Kilpatrick, K.; Donald, F.; Kaasalainen, S.; Harbman, P.; Carter, N.; Kioke, S.; et al. Advanced practice nursing in Canada: Overview of a decision support synthesis. *Nurs. Leadersh.* **2010**, *23*, 15–34. [CrossRef] [PubMed]
38. Droog, E.; Armstrong, C.; MacCurtain, S. Supporting patients during their breast cancer journey: The informational role of clinical nurse specialists. *Cancer Nurs.* **2014**, *37*, 429–435. [CrossRef]

39. World Health Organization. *Munich Declaration: Nurses and Midwives—A Force for Health*; Regional Office for Europe: Copenhagen, Denmark, 2000.
40. Aubin, M.; Giguère, A.; Martin, M.; Verreault, R.; Fitch, M.I.; Kazanjian, A.; Carmichael, P.-H. Interventions to improve continuity of care in the follow-up of patients with cancer. *Cochrane Database Syst. Rev.* **2012**, *7*, CD007672. [CrossRef]
41. Hudson, S.V.; Chubak, J.; Coups, E.J.; Blake-Gumbs, L.; Jacobsen, P.B.; Neugut, A.I.; Buist, D.S. Identifying key questions to advance research and practice in cancer survivorship follow-up care: A report from the ASPO Survivorship Interest Group. *Cancer Epidemiol. Biomarkers Prev.* **2009**, *18*, 2152–2154. [CrossRef]
42. Chen, Y.Y.; Hsieh, C.I.; Chung, K.P. Continuity of Care, Follow-Up Care, and Outcomes among Breast Cancer Survivors. *Int. J. Environ. Res. Public Health* **2019**, *16*, 3050. [CrossRef] [PubMed]
43. Skolarus, T.A.; Zhang, Y.; Hollenbeck, B.K. Understanding fragmentation of prostate cancer survivorship care: Implications for cost and quality. *Cancer* **2012**, *118*, 2837–2845. [CrossRef] [PubMed]
44. Monas, L.; Toren, O.; Uziely, B.; Chinitz, D. The oncology nurse coordinator: Role perceptions of staff members and nurse coordinators. *Isr. J. Health Policy Res.* **2017**, *6*, 66. [CrossRef]
45. Albers-Heitner, P.; Berghmans, B.; Joore, M.; Lagro-Janssen, T.; Severens, J.; Nieman, F.; Winkens, R. The effects of involving a nurse practitioner in primary care for adult patients with urinary incontinence: The PromoCon study (Promoting Continence). *BMC Health Serv. Res.* **2008**, *8*, 84. [CrossRef]
46. Horlait, M.; De Regge, M.; Baes, S.; Eeckloo, K.; Leys, M. Exploring non-physician care professionals' roles in cancer multidisciplinary team meetings: A qualitative study. *PLoS ONE* **2022**, *17*, e0263611. [CrossRef]
47. McHugh, G.A.; Horne, M.; Chalmers, K.I.; Luker, K.A. Specialist community nurses: A critical analysis of their role in the management of long-term conditions. *Int. J. Environ. Res. Public Health* **2009**, *6*, 2550–2567. [CrossRef] [PubMed]
48. Ness, E. The Oncology Clinical Research Nurse Study Co-Ordinator: Past, Present, and Future. *Asia Pac. J. Oncol. Nurs.* **2020**, *7*, 237–242. [CrossRef] [PubMed]
49. Rendle, K.A.; Abramson, C.M.; Garrett, S.B.; Halley, M.C.; Dohan, D. Beyond exploratory: A tailored framework for designing and assessing qualitative health research. *BMJ Open* **2019**, *9*, e030123. [CrossRef] [PubMed]
50. Tong, A.; Sainsbury, P.; Craig, J. Consolidated criteria for reporting qualitative research (COREQ): A 32-item checklist for interviews and focus groups. *Int. J. Qual. Health Care* **2007**, *19*, 349–357. [CrossRef]

Disclaimer/Publisher's Note: The statements, opinions and data contained in all publications are solely those of the individual author(s) and contributor(s) and not of MDPI and/or the editor(s). MDPI and/or the editor(s) disclaim responsibility for any injury to people or property resulting from any ideas, methods, instructions or products referred to in the content.

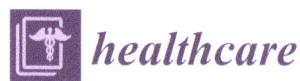 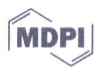

Article

Caregiving Self-Efficacy of the Caregivers of Family Members with Oral Cancer—A Descriptive Study

Ching-Hui Cheng [1], Shu-Yuan Liang [2,*], Ling Lin [1], Tzu-Ting Chang [3], Tsae-Jyy Wang [2] and Ying Lin [2]

1. Department of Nursing, Cheng Hsin General Hospital, Taipei 112, Taiwan
2. School of Nursing, National Taipei University of Nursing and Health Sciences, Taipei 112, Taiwan
3. Department of Nursing, Taipei Veterans General Hospital, Taipei 112, Taiwan
* Correspondence: shuyuan@ntunhs.edu.tw

Abstract: In Taiwan, oral cancer is the fourth most common cause of cancer death in men. The complications and side effects of oral cancer treatment pose a considerable challenge to family caregivers. The purpose of this study was to analyze the self-efficacy of the primary family caregivers of patients with oral cancer at home. A cross-sectional descriptive research design and convenience recruiting were adopted to facilitate sampling, and 107 patients with oral cancer and their primary family caregivers were recruited. The Caregiver Caregiving Self-Efficacy Scale-Oral Cancer was selected as the main instrument to be used. The primary family caregivers' mean overall self-efficacy score was 6.87 (SD = 1.65). Among all the dimensions, managing patient-related nutritional issues demonstrated the highest mean score (mean = 7.56, SD = 1.83), followed by exploring and making decisions about patient care (mean = 7.05, SD = 1.92), acquiring resources (mean = 6.89, SD = 1.80), and managing sudden and uncertain patient conditions (mean = 6.17, SD = 2.09). Our results may assist professional medical personnel to focus their educational strategies and caregiver self-efficacy enhancement strategies on the dimensions that scored relatively low.

Keywords: caregiving self-efficacy; family caregiver; oral cancer

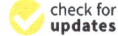

Citation: Cheng, C.-H.; Liang, S.-Y.; Lin, L.; Chang, T.-T.; Wang, T.-J.; Lin, Y. Caregiving Self-Efficacy of the Caregivers of Family Members with Oral Cancer—A Descriptive Study. *Healthcare* 2023, 11, 762. https://doi.org/10.3390/healthcare11050762

Academic Editor: Margaret Fitch

Received: 30 December 2022
Revised: 2 March 2023
Accepted: 3 March 2023
Published: 5 March 2023

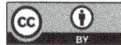

Copyright: © 2023 by the authors. Licensee MDPI, Basel, Switzerland. This article is an open access article distributed under the terms and conditions of the Creative Commons Attribution (CC BY) license (https://creativecommons.org/licenses/by/4.0/).

1. Introduction

In 2018, oral cancer incidence and death were the highest among men in Taiwan, and oral cancer was the fourth most common cause of cancer-induced death in men [1]. When patients with oral cancer undergo treatment and experience its side effects [2–4], patients themselves, their families, and medical caregivers encounter great challenges in caregiving.

Stage classification of oral cancer includes four stages according to the size of the primary tumor (T), involvement of locoregional lymph nodes (N), and distant metastases (M) [5–8]. Stage I is determined by T1–2 and N0–1, stage II by T1–2 and N2 or T3 and N0–2, and stage III by T4 or N3. Stage IV is for patients with metastatic disease [7]. This classification can aid in treatment planning, the estimation of recurrence risk, and the assessment of patient survival [5]. The overall 5-year survival rate for patients in a cohort study at Memorial Sloan Kettering Cancer Center was 63% [9]. In a multicenter retrospective analysis, an advanced T stage was significantly correlated with poor overall survival and disease-specific survival of patients [10]. Lymph node involvement is the most important prognostic factor in oral cancer. The survival rate is reduced by 50% when compared with those with similar primary tumors without neck lymph node involvement [11,12]. The impact of oral cancer at different stages on patients' physical symptoms and impairments was supported, especially the impact of advanced oral cancer [13].

Oral cancer treatment may involve the combined use of surgery, chemotherapy, and radiotherapy, among which surgery is the most essential [14]. However, surgical treatment may change patients' facial appearance and cause oral disabilities, such as impaired communication and eating functions [2]. In addition, patients with oral cancer encounter the side effects of chemotherapy or radiotherapy. Therefore, care for oral cancer is more challenging than that for other cancers [15].

In Taiwan, family members play a crucial role in the home care of patients with oral cancer, as exemplified by the trends during outpatient treatment. For instance, these family members handle patients' nutritional problems, make care decisions, manage disease-related emergencies, and seek relevant resources [16]. However, the difficulties they encounter during home care [16] may discourage these family members from putting effort into patient care, particularly when they lack belief in their own capability, worsening the subsequent care results.

Self-efficacy refers to an individual's capability belief or perceived capability to perform specific health care behavior [17]. During health care processes, self-efficacy is an essential ability that helps individuals overcome difficulties and strive for better health [18]. Self-efficacy is a key factor that affects health care behavior [19] because self-efficacy positively affects individuals' behavioral motivation and persistence when they encounter care difficulties [18].

In the research literature, investigations that examined the difference in gender regarding self-efficacy produced inconsistent findings. Several researchers described self-efficacy as one factor that accounts for gender differences [20,21]. While some researchers suggested that men reported greater self-efficacy than women [20], others suggested that females reported greater efficacy than men [21]. In contrast, no gender differences regarding self-efficacy ratings were noted in some studies [22–24].

Bandura [25] also suggested that age may be a factor that contributes to personal efficacy due to the biological processes of aging resulting in declining ability. Research on the effects of age on self-efficacy has produced mixed results [20,22–24]. Several studies indicated no relationship between self-efficacy ratings and age [20,22,24].

Educational and socio-economic levels may also be personal factors that are associated with self-efficacy since they lead to better access to resources. A researcher has suggested self-efficacy expectations as one factor that accounts for educational differences in responses to outcome measures [22]. However, several studies showed no relationship between self-efficacy and educational levels [23,24]. Most studies on the effects of economic levels on self-efficacy showed no significant difference [23,24].

Understanding the self-efficacy of family caregivers can assist medical teams to understand their capability belief in taking care of patients with oral cancer at home, identify relevant influential factors, and provide countermeasures to enhance their capability belief in patient care. This may improve the home care quality for patients with oral cancer. Therefore, the purpose of this study was to assess the self-efficacy of the primary family caregivers of patients with oral cancer at home.

2. Methods

2.1. Study Design

The current study adopted a cross-sectional descriptive research design and convenience recruiting to facilitate the sampling and discussion on the self-efficacy of the primary family caregivers of patients with oral cancer at home.

2.2. Sample and Procedure

In total, 107 primary family caregivers of outpatients were recruited for a structured questionnaire survey. The participants were enrolled from the radiology outpatient department of a teaching hospital in northern Taiwan from May 2016 to May 2018. Only patients who (1) were aged ≥20 years; (2) were diagnosed as having oral cancer; and (3) received oral cancer-related surgery, chemotherapy, or radiotherapy were included. Moreover, the family caregivers of these patients were required to be (1) aged ≥20 years, (2) recognized as the primary family caregivers by the patients, and (3) living with the patients.

After this study passed the ethical review and the family caregivers signed the informed consent form, a research assistant distributed our questionnaires to the family caregivers. The assistant checked whether the retrieved questionnaires were completely filled out immediately after the caregivers submitted them. The participants who missed items were asked to fill them out. Regarding patient medical characteristics, they were all collected from medical records by the research assistant.

2.3. Ethical Considerations

This study was approved by the institutional review board of a teaching hospital in northern Taiwan (VGHIRB No.: 2014-04-001AC). The research assistant verbally explained the research objective, data protection principles, and research procedures to obtain the participants' consent and asked them to sign the informed consent form. Codes were used in the questionnaire in place of personal information to protect participant privacy. For participants who were unwilling to proceed with the survey or were not physically suitable for further investigations, the research assistant acknowledged their withdrawal intention and stopped collecting their data.

3. Measures

3.1. Sociodemographic Variables

The current study collected the sociodemographic variables of the family caregivers and patients' medical characteristics. The collected sociodemographic variables were sex, age, marital status, education level, religious affiliation, employment status, and household income. The collected medical characteristics were the time of sickness, stage of cancer, current treatment status, and treatment side effects. Information related to the family caregivers, such as the family caregivers' relationships with the patients, manner of care, and care time, were also collected.

3.2. Caregiver Caregiving Self-Efficacy Scale-Oral Cancer

The current study applied the Caregiver Caregiving Self-Efficacy Scale-Oral Cancer (CSES-OC) [26] to estimate the self-efficacy of the family caregivers. The scale consisted of 18 items. According to factor analysis, the scale could be divided into four subscales: acquiring resources (AR; six items), managing sudden and uncertain patient conditions (MS; five items), managing patient-related nutritional issues (MN; four items), and exploring and making decisions on patient care (MD; three items). Some examples of the items for AR are "I am confident that I am able to acquire financial support", "I am confident that I am able to seek consultation on the provision of sick family member care", and "I am confident that I am able to acquire respite from caregiving". Examples for MS are "I am confident that I am able to manage the sudden onset of conditions in the sick family member", "I am confident that I am able to handle uncertainty about cancer progression", and "I am confident that I am able to handle the sick family member's uncertainty about death". Examples for MN are "I am confident that I am able to prepare a suitable diet" and "I am confident that I am able to improve the sick family member's willingness to eat". Examples of the items for MD are "I am confident that I am able to explore the most suitable care for the sick family member" and "I am confident that I am able to make decisions on sick family member care". The Cronbach's alpha of each subscale ranged between 0.78 and 0.91, and that of the overall scale was 0.95. The test–retest reliability with a 2-week interval was $r = 0.83$ ($p < 0.001$), and its criterion-related validity with the General Self-Efficacy Scale was $r = 0.59$ ($p < 0.001$). Regarding the scale used, an 11-point Likert-type scale ranging from 0 (not at all confident) to 10 (completely confident) points was adopted, where the higher the total score, the higher the self-efficacy [26].

3.3. Statistical Analysis

The current study used SPSS for Windows (version 22.0; SPSS, Chicago, IL, USA) for the data processing. Descriptive statistics, such as means, SDs, frequencies, and percentages, were obtained to examine the family caregivers' sociodemographic variables, patients' medical characteristics, caregiver–patient relationships, manner of care, care times, and caregiving self-efficacies. The differences in the variables in caregiving self-efficacy (e.g., family caregivers' sociodemographic variables, patients' medical characteristics, caregiver–patient relationships, and manner of care) were estimated using the independent sample t-test and analysis of variance (ANOVA). In addition, a Pearson product–moment correlation test was performed to verify the correlation between caregiver age, care time, patient time of sickness, and caregiving self-efficacy.

4. Results

4.1. Sociodemographic Variables of the Primary Family Caregivers and the Manner of Care

The current study recruited 107 primary family caregivers as participants, with a mean age of 51 years (SD = 10.8 years, range = 20–70 years). Among the participants, 91.6% were female, 72.9% were the patients' spouses, 56.1% had an education level of senior high school and above, 87.9% were married, 26.2% were continuing their job, 47.7% had an annual household income of <TWD 500,000, 86.9% had a religious affiliation, and 26.2% had a chronic disease (Table 1). Moreover, 41.1% provided care with the assistance of other caregivers, 40.2% provided care without rest, 83.20% had no experience in patient care, and the mean care time was 36.4 months (SD = 40.3 months, range = 1–171 months; Table 1).

Table 1. Sociodemographic variables of the primary family caregivers and the differences in overall caregiving self-efficacy between or among groups (n = 107).

Variable	Number	%	Mean	SD	t/F	p
Sex					t = −0.19	0.85
Male	9	8.4	6.77	1.40		
Female	98	91.6	6.87	1.68		
Relationship with the patient					t = −0.37	0.71
Spouse	78	72.9	6.83	1.76		
Other	29	27.1	6.96	1.37		
Education level					t = 1.52	0.13
Junior high school and below	47	43.9	7.14	1.66		
Senior high school and above	60	56.1	6.65	1.63		
Marital status					t = 0.66	0.51
Married/cohabiting	94	87.9	6.90	1.68		
Other	13	12.1	6.58	1.45		
Employment status					F = 1.25	0.30
Resigned	19	17.8	6.33	1.53		
Employed, providing care after work	28	26.2	7.05	1.52		
Employed, on leave	11	10.3	6.45	1.72		
Other	49	45.8	7.06	1.74		
Annual household income (in TWD)					F = 0.13	0.88
<500,000	51	47.7	6.80	1.59		
510,000–1,000,000	39	36.4	6.88	1.79		
>1,010,000	17	15.9	7.03	1.61		
Religious affiliation					t = 1.32	0.19
Yes	93	86.9	6.95	1.63		
No	14	13.1	6.32	1.79		
Chronic disease					t = 0.01	0.99
Yes	28	26.2	6.86	1.78		
No	79	73.8	6.87	1.62		
Manner of care					F = 1.16	0.32
With the assistance of other caregivers	44	41.1	7.16	1.56		
Independent, full-day care	28	26.2	6.63	1.93		
Independent, non-full-day care	35	32.7	6.69	1.52		
Weekly care time					F = 0.24	0.78

Table 1. Cont.

Variable	Number	%	Mean	SD	t/F	p
Without rest	43	40.2	6.88	1.77		
With weekly rest time	24	22.4	7.04	1.65		
With irregular rest time	40	37.4	6.74	1.55		
Past care experience					t = 1.02	0.31
Yes	18	16.8	6.50	1.48		
No	89	83.2	6.94	1.69		

4.2. Patients' Medical Characteristics

Among the 107 patients with oral cancer, the mean time of sickness was 42.5 months (SD = 44.4 months, range = 1–171 months). Of all the patients, 36.4% had stage IV oral cancer, 78.5% had completed their treatment, and 36.4% were still experiencing the side effects of the treatment (Table 2).

4.3. Caregiving Self-Efficacy of the Primary Family Caregivers

The CSES-OC was used to measure the self-efficacy of the primary family caregivers. The overall and subscale (i.e., AR, MS, MN, and MD) scores were considered. The mean overall self-efficacy score was 6.87 (SD = 1.65). Moreover, of all the subscales, MN demonstrated the highest mean score of 7.56 (SD = 1.83), followed by MD (7.05, SD = 1.92), AR (6.89, SD = 1.80), and MS (6.17, SD = 2.09) (Table 3).

Table 2. Patients' medical characteristics and the differences in overall caregiving self-efficacy between or among groups ($n = 107$).

Variable	Number	%	Mean	SD	t/F	p
Stage of cancer					F = 0.50	0.68
Stage I	22	20.6	7.00	2.09		
Stage II	32	29.9	6.59	1.55		
Stage III	14	13.1	7.16	1.81		
Stage IV	39	36.4	6.91	1.43		
Current treatment status					t = 0.79	0.43
Receiving treatment	23	21.5	6.62	1.67		
Not receiving treatment	84	78.5	6.93	1.65		
Side effects					t = 0.84	0.40
Yes	39	36.4	6.69	1.60		
No	68	63.6	6.97	1.69		

Table 3. Caregiving self-efficacy in primary family caregivers ($n = 107$).

Variable	Mean	SD	Minimum	Maximum
Acquiring resources (AR)	6.89	1.80	1.50	10.00
Managing sudden and uncertain patient conditions (MS)	6.17	2.09	1.00	10.00
Managing patient-related nutritional issues (MN)	7.56	1.83	1.75	10.00
Exploring and making decisions on patient care (MD)	7.05	1.92	2.00	10.00
Total self-efficacy	6.87	1.65	2.00	10.00

4.4. Differences in the Sociodemographic Variables of the Primary Family Caregivers and Manner of Care in Caregiving Self-Efficacy

No significant correlations were discovered between the overall self-efficacy score and age ($r = 0.06$, $p > 0.05$) and between the overall self-efficacy score and care time ($r = 0.08$, $p > 0.05$). Moreover, no significant differences were noted for the other sociodemographic variables and manner of care in caregiving self-efficacy (Table 1).

4.5. Differences in Medical Characteristics in Caregiving Self-Efficacy

No significant correlations were discovered between the time of sickness and the overall self-efficacy score ($r = 0.11$, $p > 0.05$). Moreover, the differences among patients' other medical characteristics in the overall self-efficacy were nonsignificant (Table 2).

5. Discussion

In this study, the researchers analyzed the caregiving self-efficacy of the primary family caregivers of patients with oral cancer. Results of the current study may aid professional caregivers in understanding the capability belief of primary family caregivers in facing challenges during the care process and the most challenging tasks they are likely to encounter.

According to the self-efficacy classification proposed by Kobau and DiIorio [27], a self-efficacy score of 4–7 (range: 0–10) denotes a moderate level of self-efficacy. Here, the mean caregiving self-efficacy score was 6.87, indicating that the caregivers in this study had moderate self-efficacy. However, because the scoring methods used for measuring self-efficacy have varied between previous relevant studies [28–30], the researchers could not compare the results of the current study with those of other studies directly. The mean self-efficacy score of the current study was close to that of Liang, Yates, Edwards, and Tsay [22], where the opioid-taking self-efficacy of patients with cancer was estimated, and it was slightly lower than that of Kobau and DiIorio [27], where the self-efficacy of patients with epilepsy was assessed. The possible reason for this was that the care difficulty differed between diseases, which may have affected the participants' perceived level of capability.

Here, the caregiving self-efficacy in the MN dimension scored the highest, with a mean score of 7.56. Handling the nutritional issues of patients might not be the most challenging task for caregivers. Increasing their willingness to eat and preparing suitable food for them [26] were found to be essential behavior tasks to promote their physiological recovery.

The self-efficacy in the MD dimension scored the second highest, with a mean score of 7.05. In this dimension, the behavior tasks relevant to caregiving self-efficacy included managing the side effects due to cancer treatment and making treatment-related decisions [26]. These types of behavior tasks aim at providing home-based medical assistance.

Moreover, the AR dimension scored the third highest, with a mean score of 6.89. Here, the caregiving self-efficacy-related behavior tasks encompass managing emotional issues, receiving care counseling, and being able to rest during the care process [26]. Emotional management was related to tasks such as dealing with the emotions of patients who were facing oral cancer treatment and prognosis, as well as the emotions of caregivers themselves [16,26]. According to the current results, this was the second most challenging set of behavioral tasks. It was a self-assistance behavior task related to the maintenance of the physical and mental health of the caregivers themselves.

Finally, the MS dimension scored the lowest, with a mean score of 6.17. For caregivers, handling the safety and death issues of patients was the most challenging task. The caregiving self-efficacy-related behavior tasks include handling sudden situations, managing the uncertainty in the disease process, and managing poor prognosis [26]. These most difficult care tasks indicate the care priorities for patients and their family caregivers for health care professionals.

Family caregivers' capability belief (i.e., self-efficacy) is a key factor that affects subsequent care behavior and care results [31,32]. Professional medical personnel can increase family caregivers' capability belief according to the four sources of efficacy beliefs in the self-efficacy theory: family caregivers' performance accomplishment, vicarious experience, professional caregivers' verbal persuasion, and consideration of family caregivers' physical and emotional arousal [17,32]. Furthermore, professional medical personnel could integrate relevant educational strategies, including diary logs [33], videos, and brochures [32], to improve family caregivers' capability beliefs in taking care of patients with oral cancer.

In this study, the researchers adopted a cross-sectional descriptive research design. Therefore, the current study could not obtain the changes in family caregiving self-efficacy with respect to the patient's condition or required care time. The present study involved all patients in the disease period. The timing of patient enrollment was not controlled. Some patients were still undergoing their course of treatment, some patients had finished their treatment. Different times or stages of treatment may affect the challenge of the care of family and, therefore, may affect their ability cognition. In addition, the sample size was small for all sociodemographic and medical variable groups. It is unlikely that statistical differences could be detected in this population. On the other hand, the current research used convenience sampling, which may have caused sampling deviation. Families with large care loads may have been eliminated naturally. The samples were collected from a teaching hospital in northern Taiwan alone, which might affect the inference of the current results.

6. Conclusions

Our current results indicated that family caregiving self-efficacy scores in the CSES-OC MS and AR items were the lowest and the second lowest, respectively. The current study recommends that professional medical teams focus their educational strategies and caregiver self-efficacy enhancement strategies on the dimensions that scored relatively low (i.e., handling patients' safety and death issues and managing physical and mental health problems through self-assistance). For example, issues in these dimensions include managing the emotional distress of a sick family member and the caregiver themself, handling uncertainty about the sick family member's cancer progression and death, and managing the sudden onset of conditions in the sick family member. Through family caregivers' performance accomplishment, vicarious experience, professional caregivers' verbal persuasion, consideration of caregivers' physical and emotional arousal, and using educational media, the self-efficacy of family caregivers regarding taking care of a patient with cancer may be increased. The current results are from an exploratory study. The cut-off point of the self-efficacy score in this study refers to the research results of other patient groups. The current study suggests that more studies are needed.

Author Contributions: Conceptualization and methodology: C.-H.C. and S.-Y.L.; investigation: T.-T.C., L.L. and Y.L.; data curation: T.-T.C.; formal analysis and data curation: C.-H.C., S.-Y.L. and T.-J.W.; writing—original draft preparation: S.-Y.L., writing—review and editing: T.-J.W.; funding acquisition: C.-H.C., S.-Y.L. and L.L.; supervision and project administration: C.-H.C. and S.-Y.L. All authors have read and agreed to the published version of the manuscript.

Funding: This research was funded by the Cheng Hsin General Hospital, grant number CHGH111-(IU)08 and the APC was funded by CHGH111- (IU)08.

Institutional Review Board Statement: The study was conducted in accordance with the Declaration of Helsinki, and approved by the Institutional Review Board of Taipei Veterans General Hospital (protocol code 2014-04-001 AC and date of approval: 5 May 2014).

Informed Consent Statement: Informed consent was obtained from all subjects involved in the study.

Data Availability Statement: The data presented in this study are available from the corresponding author upon reasonable request.

Conflicts of Interest: The authors declare no conflict of interest.

References

1. Ministry of Health and Welfare. Cancer Registry Annual Report. 2018. Available online: https://www.hpa.gov.tw/Pages/Detail.aspx?nodeid=269&pid=13498 (accessed on 7 April 2022).
2. Gobbo, M.; Bullo, F.; Perinetti, G.; Gatto, A.; Ottaviani, G.; Biasotto, M.; Tirelli, G. Diagnostic and therapeutic features associated with modification of quality-of-life's outcomes between one and six months after major surgery for head and neck cancer. *Braz. J. Otorhinolaryngol.* **2016**, *82*, 548–557. [CrossRef]

3. Pedersen, B.; Koktved, D.P.; Nielsen, L.L. Living with side effects from cancer treatment—A challenge to target information. *Scand. J. Caring Sci.* **2013**, *27*, 715–723. [CrossRef]
4. Semple, C.J.; Dunwoody, L.; Kernohan, W.G. Changes and challenges to patients' lifestyle patterns following treatment for head and neck cancer. *J. Adv. Nurs.* **2008**, *63*, 85–93. [CrossRef] [PubMed]
5. Almangush, A.; Mäkitie, A.A.; Triantafyllou, A.; de Bree, R.; Strojan, P.; Rinaldo, A.; Hernandez-Prera, J.C.; Suárez, C.; Kowalski, L.P.; Ferlito, A.; et al. Staging and grading of oral squamous cell carcinoma: An update. *Oral Oncol.* **2020**, *107*, 104799. [CrossRef]
6. Lydiatt, W.M.; Patel, S.G.; O'Sullivan, B.; Brandwein, M.S.; Ridge, J.A.; Migliacci, J.C.; Loomis, A.M.; Shah, J.P. Head and Neck Cancers—Major Changes in the American Joint Committee on Cancer Eighth Edition Cancer Staging Manual. *CA Cancer J. Clin.* **2017**, *67*, 122–137. [CrossRef] [PubMed]
7. Glastonbury, C.M. Critical Changes in the Staging of Head and Neck Cancer. *Radiol. Imaging Cancer* **2020**, *2*, e190022. [CrossRef] [PubMed]
8. Wong, T.S.C.; Wiesenfeld, D. Oral Cancer. *Aust. Dent. J.* **2018**, *63*, S91–S99. [CrossRef]
9. Zanoni, D.K.; Montero, P.H.; Migliacci, J.C.; Shah, J.P.; Wong, R.J.; Ganly, I.; Patel, S.G. Survial outcomes after treatment of cancer of the oral cavity (1985–2015). *Oral Oncol.* **2019**, *90*, 115–121. [CrossRef] [PubMed]
10. Sakamoto, Y.; Otsuru, M.; Hasegawa, T.; Akashi, M.; Yamada, S.; Kurita, H.; Okura, M.; Yamakawa, N.; Kirita, T.; Yanamoto, S.; et al. Treatment and Prognosis of Oral Cancer Patients with Confirmed Contralateral Neck Metastasis: A Multicenter Retrospective Analysis. *Int. J. Environ. Res. Public Health* **2022**, *19*, 9229. [CrossRef] [PubMed]
11. Shah, J.P.; Andersen, P.E. Evolving role of modifications in neck dissection for oral squamous carcinoma. *Br. J. Oral Maxillofac. Surg.* **1995**, *33*, 3–8. [CrossRef]
12. Robbins, K.T.; Ferlito, A.; Shah, J.P.; Hamoir, M.; Takes, R.P.; Strojan, P.; Khafif, A.; Silver, C.E.; Rinaldo, A.; Medina, J.E. The evolving role of selective neck dissection for head and neck squamous cell carcinoma. *Eur. Arch. Oto-Rhino-Laryngol. Off. J. Eur. Fed. Oto-Rhino-Laryngol. Soc.* **2013**, *270*, 1195–1202. [CrossRef]
13. Vilarim, R.C.B.; Tavares, M.R.; de Siqueira, S.R.D.T.; Jales, S.M.D.C.P.; Formigoni, G.G.S.; Teixeira, M.J.; de Siqueira, J.T.T. Characteristics and prevalence of orofacial pain as an initial symptom of oral and oropharyngeal cancer and its impact on the patient's functionality and quality of life. *Oral Surg. Oral Med. Oral Pathol. Oral Radiol.* **2022**, *134*, 457–464. [CrossRef]
14. Lin, M.C.; Leu, Y.S.; Chiang, C.J.; Ko, J.Y.; Wang, C.P.; Yang, T.L.; Chen, T.C.; Chen, C.N.; Chen, H.L.; Liao, C.T.; et al. Adequate surgical margins for oral cancer: A Taiwan cancer registry national database analysis. *Oral Oncol.* **2021**, *119*, 1053582021. [CrossRef] [PubMed]
15. Kuo, C.Y.; Liang, S.Y.; Tsay, S.L.; Wang, T.J.; Cheng, S.F. Symptom Management Tasks and Behaviors related to Chemotherapy in Taiwanese Outpatients with Breast Cancer. *Eur. J. Oncol. Nurs.* **2015**, *19*, 654–659. [CrossRef]
16. Liang, S.Y.; Chang, T.T.; Wu, W.W.; Wang, T.J. Caring for patients with oral cancer in Taiwan: The challenges faced by family caregivers. *Eur. J. Oncol. Nurs.* **2019**, *28*, e12891. [CrossRef] [PubMed]
17. Bandura, A. *Self-Efficacy: The Exercise of Control*; WH Freeman: New York, NY, USA, 1997.
18. Bandura, A. Health promotion by social cognitive means. *Health Educ. Behav.* **2004**, *31*, 143–164. [CrossRef]
19. Chin, C.H.; Tseng, L.H.; Chao, T.C.; Wang, T.J.; Wu, S.F.; Liang, S.Y. Self-Care as a Mediator between Symptom-Management Self-Efficacy and Quality of Life in Women with Breast Cancer. *PLoS ONE* **2021**, *16*, e0246430. [CrossRef]
20. Jackson, T.; Iezzi, T.; Gunderson, J.; Nagasaka, T.; Fritch, A. Gender differences in pain perception: The mediating role of self-efficacy beliefs. *Sex Roles* **2002**, *47*, 561. [CrossRef]
21. Porter, L.S.; Keefe, F.J.; McBride, C.M.; Pollak, K.; Fish, L.; Garst, J. Perceptions of patients' self-efficacy for managing pain and lung cancer symptoms: Correspondence between patients and family caregivers. *Pain* **2002**, *98*, 169–178. [CrossRef]
22. Liang, S.Y.; Yates, P.; Edwards, H.; Tsay, S.L. Opioid-taking self-efficacy amongst Taiwanese outpatients with cancer. *Support. Care Cancer* **2012**, *20*, 199–206. [CrossRef] [PubMed]
23. Al-Harithy, F.M.; Wazqar, D.Y. Factors associated with self-management practices and self-efficacy among adults with cancer under treatment in Saudi Arabia. *J. Clin. Nurs.* **2021**, *30*, 3301–3313. [CrossRef] [PubMed]
24. Ozkaraman, A.; Uzgor, F.; Dugum, O.; Peker, S. The Effect of Health Literacy on Self-Efficacy and Quality of Life among Turkish Cancer Patients. *J. Pak. Med. Assoc.* **2019**, *69*, 995–999. [PubMed]
25. Bandura, A. Self-efficacy. In *Encyclopedia of Human Behaviour*; Ramachaudran, V.S., Ed.; Academic Press: San Diego, CA, USA, 1994.
26. Cheng, J.C.; Chang, T.T.; Wang, L.W.; Liang, S.Y.; Hsu, S.C.; Wu, S.F.; Wang, T.J.; Liu, C.Y. Development and Psychometric Evaluation of the Caregiver Caregiving Self-Efficacy Scale for Family Members with Oral Cancer. *Int. J. Nurs. Pract.* **2021**, *13*, e12957. [CrossRef] [PubMed]
27. Kobau, R.; DiIorio, C. Epilepsy self-management: A comparison of self-efficacy and outcome expectancy for medication adherence and lifestyle behaviours among people with epilepsy. *Epilepsy Behav.* **2003**, *4*, 217–225. [CrossRef]
28. Augustinavicius, J.L.; Murray, S.M.; Familiar-Lopez, I.; Boivin, M.J.; Mutebe, A.; Arima, E.; Bass, J.K. Measurement of Parenting Self-efficacy Among Female HIV-Affected Caregivers in Uganda. *Matern. Child Health J.* **2020**, *24*, 319–327. [CrossRef]
29. Chyung, S.Y.; LePiane, J.; Shamsy, J.; Radloff, M. Improving caregivers' confidence with the Powerful Tools for Caregivers program. *Educ. Gerontol.* **2018**, *44*, 572–585. [CrossRef]
30. Hendrix, C.C.; Landerman, R.; Abernethy, A.P. Effects of an Individualized Caregiver Training Intervention on Self- Efficacy of Cancer Caregivers. *West. J. Nurs. Res.* **2011**, *35*, 590–610. [CrossRef]

31. Ezgi, K. The effect of a self-management program on hand-washing/mask-wearing behaviours and self-efficacy level in peritoneal dialysis patients: A pilot study. *J. Ren. Care.* **2019**, *45*, 93–101.
32. Wu, S.F.; Liang, S.Y.; Wang, T.J.; Chen, M.H.; Jian, Y.M.; Zheng, G.Z. A self-management intervention to improve quality of life and psychosocial impact for people with type 2 diabetes. *J. Clin. Nurs.* **2011**, *20*, 2655–2665. [CrossRef]
33. van der Laar, K.E.W.; van der Bijl, J.J. The theory and measurement of the self-efficacy construct. *Sch. Inq. Nurs. Pract. Int. J.* **2001**, *15*, 189–207.

Disclaimer/Publisher's Note: The statements, opinions and data contained in all publications are solely those of the individual author(s) and contributor(s) and not of MDPI and/or the editor(s). MDPI and/or the editor(s) disclaim responsibility for any injury to people or property resulting from any ideas, methods, instructions or products referred to in the content.

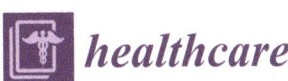

Systematic Review

The Role of Nurse on the Treatment Decision Support for Older People with Cancer: A Systematic Review

Hiroko Komatsu [1],* and Yasuhiro Komatsu [2]

1. Japanese Red Cross Kyushu International College of Nursing, 1-1 Asty, Munakata-City 811-4157, Fukuoka, Japan
2. Department of Healthcare Quality and Safety, Gunma University Graduate School of Medicine, 3-39-22 Showa-machi, Maebashi 371-8511, Gunma, Japan
* Correspondence: h-komatsu@jrckicn.ac.jp; Tel.: +81-940-35-7001

Abstract: Background: The number of older adults with cancer is increasing worldwide. The role of nurses in supporting patients' decision-making is expanding, as this process is fraught with complexity and uncertainty due to comorbidities, frailty, cognitive decline, etc., in older adults with cancer. The aim of this review was to examine the contemporary roles of oncology nurses in the treatment decision-making process in older adults with cancer. **Methods**: A systematic review of PubMed, CINAHL, and PsycINFO databases was conducted in accordance with PRISMA guidelines. **Results**: Of the 3029 articles screened, 56 full texts were assessed for eligibility, and 13 were included in the review. We identified three themes regarding nurses' roles in the decision-making process for older adults with cancer: accurate geriatric assessments, provision of available information, and advocacy. Nurses conduct geriatric assessments to identify geriatric syndromes, provide appropriate information, elicit patient preferences, and communicate efficiently with patients and caregivers, promoting physicians. Time constraints were cited as a barrier to fulfilling nurses' roles. **Conclusions**: The role of nurses is to elicit patients' broader health and social care needs to facilitate patient-centered decision-making, respecting their preferences and values. Further research focusing on the role of nurses that considers diverse cancer types and healthcare systems is needed.

Keywords: older adults; cancer; decision-making; nurse

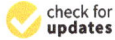

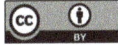

1. Introduction

Population aging has substantially contributed to an increasing number of new cancer cases worldwide [1]. The global cancer burden is expected to be 28.4 million cases in 2040, a 47% rise from 2020 [2]. The number of new cancer cases among older adults (aged 65 years and older) is expected to double by 2035 (14 million) [1]. Age is a risk factor for cancer due to the duration of carcinogenesis, the vulnerability of aging tissues to environmental carcinogens, and other bodily changes that favor the development and the growth of cancer [3].

Healthcare providers (HCPs) involved in the treatment of older adults with cancer face many challenges. Older adults with cancer often have age-related frailty [4,5], co-morbidities [6,7], and polypharmacy [8,9], which complicate the cancer diagnosis and create uncertainty in decisions about treatment goals and outcomes [7]. In addition, the involvement of caregivers and other key persons in decision-making affects the decision structure and process [10,11]. Thus, clinical practice guidelines for older patients with cancer provide recommendations for the appropriate implementation of validated and standardized clinical assessment tools and decision-making models for this vulnerable and prevalent demographic group [12]. However, over 50% of older patients with advanced cancer experience severe toxicity during the first 3 months of chemotherapy [13]. In managing cancer drug-related adverse effects and the quality of life, assessment of the values and preferences of older adults with cancer is critical to informed treatment decision-making [14].

In recent years, there has been growing evidence that geriatric assessments (GAs) can be used to assess and manage the vulnerability of older adults with cancer [7,14], and can aid in shared decision-making (SDM) regarding treatment and interventions among patients, caregivers, and oncologists [12]. Nurses are at the frontline in the care of patients with cancer, particularly in this new era of SDM [15]. Advanced nurse practitioners play a pivotal role in determining and facilitating the preferences of patients with cancer [16]. The nursing role during cancer SDM can be complicated and requires flexibility [17]. Although the importance of nurses' roles has been discussed, a synthesis of the roles of nurses in the treatment decision-making process of older adults with cancer and their effects is lacking. Therefore, this systematic review examined the contemporary roles of oncology nurses throughout the cancer treatment decision-making process of older adults with cancer.

2. Methods

2.1. Search Question

What roles do oncology nurses play in the treatment decision-making process of older adults with cancer?

2.2. Search Strategy

This review was based on a systematic, comprehensive search of three databases, including CINAHL, PubMed (via MEDLINE), and PsycINFO, and was conducted in accordance with PRISMA guidelines [18]. Manual searches of reference lists and gray literature were also performed to identify relevant articles. Searches were limited to articles published in English, database inception to September 2022. To address the research question, a broad range of key search terms based on the MeSH (Medical Subject Headings) topics of "decision making", "older adults", "cancer", and "nurse" were used. For other MESH terms, and a combination of free-text searches refer to Supplementary Files S1 and S2.

2.3. Eligibility Criteria

The literature searches aimed to identify qualitative, quantitative, and mixed-method studies that provided a description of the roles of the nurse throughout the treatment decision-making process for older adults with cancer. Studies were limited to those that focused on adults ≥ 60 years of age. Additionally, reviews, letters, case studies, editorials, and conference abstracts were excluded.

2.4. Quality Appraisal

Two reviewers (H.K. and Y.K.) discussed and selected the articles to be included in this review. Studies were selected using a two-step process. Articles were first screened by title and abstract to determine their relevance to the search question. The PRISMA search strategy [18] was used to filter articles and remove duplicates. Full-text articles were then retrieved and independently reviewed to determine whether the inclusion criteria were met. Two researchers (H.K. and Y.K.) independently evaluated the studies that met the inclusion criteria for methodological quality using the Mixed Methods Appraisal Tool (MMAT), V.2018 [19].

2.5. Thematic Analysis

We provided a narrative summary by conducting a qualitative synthesis to identify key themes based on thematic analysis [20]. First, free line-by-line coding of findings from included studies was conducted into related field. Next, thematic analysis was undertaken to construct themes related to the research questions across studies.

3. Results

A total of 3029 articles were identified through database searches supplemented by manual searches. Of these, 534 duplicates were removed; studies that were unclear on the involvement of nurses in decision support or did not focus on decision support in patients with cancer, such as those focused on cancer screening, cancer healthcare system, and treatment decisions among physicians, were excluded. Studies that focused on pediatric oncology patients were also excluded because they did not meet inclusion criteria. The remaining articles underwent full-text review and 13 were deemed suitable for inclusion (Figure 1).

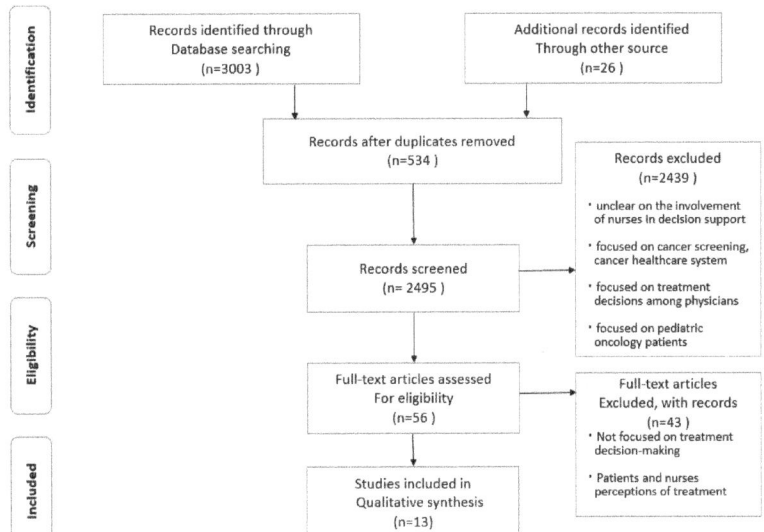

Figure 1. PRISMA flow diagram.

3.1. Study Characteristics

Table 1 presents the main characteristics of the 13 studies included in this review. Seven studies were conducted in European countries [21–27], and six in the USA or Canada [28–33]. Two studies used a quantitative cross-sectional design [22,24], one used a retrospective cohort design [26], one used a quasi-experimental design (pre-post study design) [32], one used a mixed-method design [28], six used a qualitative design [21,23,25,27,30,31], and two were case studies [29,33]. Only one study examined the effect of a nurse-led GA on treatment modifications and outcomes [26]. One pre-post study examined the effect of a Communication Skills Training module on the HCP's SDM approach to meetings with older adults with cancer and their family [32]. Two case studies described the usefulness of nursing practices in the treatment decision-making of older adults with cancer [29,33]. One quantitative cross-sectional study examined the perception of HCPs (including nurses) on treatment decisions of older adults with cancer [24]. One cross-sectional questionnaire survey investigated older women's preferences for receiving information about breast cancer treatment options [22]. Qualitative studies focused on perceptions in older adults with cancer and their partners' decision-making [30], and the perceptions of older adults with cancer [31], HCPs [21,27], and older adults with cancer, their families, and HCPs [23,25].

Table 1. Studies included in the review.

Author(s) and Year of Publication	Study Population and Setting	Objective(s)	Design	Methods	Summary of Themes	MMAT Score, %
Tariman et al. (2014) [28]	Twenty older adults (60 years of age and older) with symptomatic myeloma diagnosed within the past six months. Recruited from the Seattle Cancer Care Alliance (SCCA) or the Northwestern University Myeloma Program (NUMP), USA.	To examine patient perspectives on their personal and contextual factors relevant to treatment decision-making. The second aim was to describe physician perspectives on the treatment-decision making in older adults diagnosed with symptomatic multiple myeloma.	Quantitative. Cross sectional study. Qualitaive.	Semi-structured face-to-face interviews. Descriptive statistics and Triangulation of Qualitative and Quantitative Data.	(1) Disclosure of treatment options to patients. (2) Encouraging patients to express their decisional role preference to the physician. (3) Developing a culture of mutual respect and value the patient's desire for autonomy for treatment decision-making. (4) Acknowledging that the right to make a treatment choice belongs to the patient.	100
Bridges et al. (2015) [21]	Healthcare professionals ($n = 22$; $n = 11$ nurse specialists; $n = 11$ physician) Recruited from five English NHS hospital trusts in UK.	To investigate how cancer treatment decisions are formulated for older people with complex health and social care needs and the factors that shape these processes.	Qualitative.	Semi-structured face-to-face interviews. Framework Analysis.	(1) Giving patients quality, availability and timeliness of information and opportunities for discussion. (2) Attention of complex patient-centred information and preference in the meeting. (3) Advocating for the patient's autonomy and right to make informed decisions. (4) Involved in multidisciplinary teams focus on complex patient-centered information, such as comorbidities, psychosocial and supportive care needs, and patient preferences.	100

Table 1. *Cont.*

Author(s) and Year of Publication	Study Population and Setting	Objective(s)	Design	Methods	Summary of Themes	MMAT Score, %
Burton et al. (2017) [22]	Women, ≥75 years, who had been offered a choice between PET and surgery at diagnosis of breast cancer. (n = 101) Recruited from 10 NHS breast units across England and Wales.	To further establish older women's preferences regarding receiving information about breast cancer treatment options (surgery or PET) and quantify issues raised in the interview study. To quantify women's preferences regarding the presentation of information and establish their preferred decision-making styles.	Quantitative. Cross sectional study.	Multicentre survey using questionaire. Descriptive statistics.	(1) Ensuring that women receive the preferred level and amount of information as well as involvement when making treatment decisions. (2) Help patients reach their preferred level of information and involvement in decision making using decision support tools.	100
Shahrokni et al. (2017) [29]	An 88-years old patient with colon cancer. Recruited from Cancer Center, USA.	To describe how the Geriatrics Service at Cancer Center approaches an older patient with colon cancer from presentation to the end of life, show the importance of geriatric assessment at the various stages of cancer treatment, and how predictive models are used to tailor the treatment.	Qualitative. Case Study Design.	Retrospective case.	(1) Perform geriatric assessment and identify geriatric syndromes. (2) Manage comorbid conditions that could prevent successful cancer treatment. (3) Effectively and efficiently communicate with patient and caregivers, oncologist, and primary care physician.	-

Table 1. *Cont.*

Author(s) and Year of Publication	Study Population and Setting	Objective(s)	Design	Methods	Summary of Themes	MMAT Score, %
Jones et al. (2018) [30]	Thirty-five pairs of patients and their decision partners (16 pairs reflected patients with less than 6 months since their diagnosis of metastatic castration-resistant prostate cancer). Recruited from Cancer Center, USA.	To describe and understand the lived experience of patients with advanced prostate cancer and their decision partners who utilized an interactive decision aid to make informed, shared treatment decisions.	Qualitative.	Semi-structured interview. Hermeneutic phenomenological approach.	(1) Facilitating to discuss issues thoroughly between patients and decision partners by using decision aids. (2) Facilitating closer patient-healthcare provider relationships by using decision aids.	100
McWilliams (2018) [23]	Patients with a diagnosis of cancer-dementia ($n = 10$), informal caregivers ($n = 9$), and oncology HCPs ($n = 12$). Recruited from a regional treatment cancer centre, UK.	To explore the cancer-related information needs and decision-making experiences of patients with cancer and comorbid dementia, their informal caregivers, and oncology healthcare professionals.	Qualitative. Cross-sectional study.	Semi-structured face-to-face interviews. Thematic analysis.	(1) Communicating clinically relevant information. (2) Suggesting that dementia-related cognitive and communication impairments influence treatment options in relation to potential side effects and appropriate management. (3) Navigating treatment decision-making information.	100
Sattar et al. (2018) [31]	Ten patients aged ≥ 65 in the curative/palliative setting (presenting with breast, prostate, colorectal, or lung cancer) and who had made a treatment decision in the preceding six months. A Cancer Centre, University Health Network or Health Sciences Centre, Toronto, Ontario, Canada.	To explore the factors that were important for accepting or refusing cancer treatment by older adults undergoing chemotherapy and/or radiation therapy.	Qualitative.	Semi-structured face-to-face interviews. Framework Analysis.	(1) Coaching patients on how to seek evidence-based discussion regarding treatment options. (2) Providing supplementary education on treatment options.	100

Table 1. *Cont.*

Author(s) and Year of Publication	Study Population and Setting	Objective(s)	Design	Methods	Summary of Themes	MMAT Score, %
de Augst et al. (2019) [24]	Health care providers ($n = 170$), including 82 urologists, 31 oncologists, and 57 oncology nurses. Recruited from participants of meeting of the Netherlands Association for Urology and urologists and oncology nurses by the Netherlands Association for Urology and Dutch National Consultation Oncology Nurses, Netherlands.	To evaluate perspectives of the multidisciplinary team concerning shared decision-making in treatment decisions for older patients with metastatic castration-resistant prostate cancer.	Quantitative. Cross sectional study.	A validated survey using questionnaire. Descriptive statistics	(1) Elicit individual patient preferences using Decision-Aids. (2) Offer patients the opportunity to gain knowledge about their disease and values in their own time with their family.	100
Griffiths et al. (2020) [25]	Seventeen people with dementia and cancer, twenty-two relatives, and nineteen staff members (Clinical nurse specialists; $n = 8$). Recruited from Oncology and associated departments in two National Health Service (NHS) Trusts in one UK region and their local communities.	To explore cancer decision-making experiences of people with cancer and dementia, their families, and healthcare staff.	Qualitative.	Semi-structured interview. Ethnographically informed thematic analysis.	(1) Ensure people with cancer and dementia apply an individualized ability focused assessment. (2) Consider which options were appropriate for patients based on multiple factors.	100

Table 1. *Cont.*

Author(s) and Year of Publication	Study Population and Setting	Objective(s)	Design	Methods	Summary of Themes	MMAT Score, %
Shen et al. (2020) [32]	Health care providers (n = 99), 24 advance practice providers (including nurse practitioners and physician assistants); 23 nurses, 14 social workers, 13 physicians, and 20 other health care providers. Recruited from community-based centers, cancer centers, and hospitals in the Northeastern U.S.	To evaluate a Communication Skills Training (CST) module for health care providers applying a shared decision-making approach to a meeting with an older adult with cancer and his/her family.	Quantitative. Pre/post study design.	Pre- and post-training Standardized Patient Assessments and a survey on their confidence in and intent to utilize skills taught. Descriptive statistics.	(1) Improve collaborative shared decision making among providers, patients, and family members in the context of older adults with cancer. (2) Promote an active dialogue between the triad while respecting patient values and preferences.	75
Strohschein et al. (2020) [33]	An 89-year-old man with head and neck cancer. Recruited from Cancer Center in Toronto, Canada.	To present comprehensive geriatric assessment (CGA) as an approach to personalizing care for older adults with cancer.	Qualitative. Case Study Design.	Retrospective case. describe the process of CGA and an overview of geriatric oncology screening and assessment.	(1) Integrate geriatric assessment tools into practice to identify and address age-related concerns. (2) Facilitate communication and contribute to personalization of care. (3) Spent a time on patient assessments during the decision-making process.	-
Festen et al. (2021) [26]	Two hundred fourteen patients with cancer of 70 years and older were primarily seen at the surgical outpatient clinic. Recruited from a University Medical Center, Netherlands.	A novel care pathway was set up incorporating geriatric assessment into treatment decision-making for older cancer patients. Treatment decisions could be modified following discussion in an onco-geriatric multidisciplinary team (MDT). To assess the effect of treatment modifications on outcomes.	Quantitative. Retrospective study.	Retrospective analysis of outcomes. Descriptive statistics.	(1) Incorporating nurse-led geriatric assessment in decision-making. (2) Assess the patient preferences regarding treatment outcomes. (3) Spent a time on patient assessments during the decision-making process.	100

Table 1. *Cont.*

Author(s) and Year of Publication	Study Population and Setting	Objective(s)	Design	Methods	Summary of Themes	MMAT Score, %
Dijkman et al. (2022) [27]	Thirteen surgeons and thirteen nurses. Recruited from two hospitals in the northern Netherlands.	To explore how surgeons and nurses perceive the involvement of adult children of older patients with cancer in treatment decision-making.	Qualitative.	Open in-depth interviews. Thematic analysis.	(1) Ensure positive family involvement in treatment decision-making. (2) Stimulate the communication and deliberation between patients and their adult children.	100

3.2. Quality Assessment

Among the 13 included studies, two were case studies and did not undergo quality assessment; the remaining 11 primary studies underwent methodological quality assessment using the MMAT [19]. These studies met 100% of the quality criteria, with the exception of one study that met 75% of the quality criteria, and had high quality scores (Table 1, Supplementary File S3).

3.3. Themes of Included Studies

The data were categorized into three themes regarding the nurse's role in the treatment decision-making process of older adults with cancer: (a) accurate GAs, (b) provision of available information, and (c) advocacy.

3.4. Accurate GAs

The oncology nurse plays an important role in assessing the factors to be considered in the cancer treatment decision-making process by properly implementing GAs in older adults with cancer. Festen et al. conducted a retrospective analysis of the outcomes of nurse-led GAs and patient preference assessment; they found that nurse-led GAs may lead to the tailoring of treatment decisions to the patient's frailty status and preferences, and improve outcomes [26]. There was no significant difference in one-year mortality between the unchanged and modified group (29.7% versus 26.1%, $p = 0.7$). There were, however, significantly fewer days spent in hospital (median 5 vs. 8.5 days $p = 0.02$) and fewer grade II or higher postoperative complications (13.3% versus 35.5% $p = 0.005$) in the modified group. Additionally, two case studies reported on the usefulness of advanced practice nurses. Specifically, Shahrokni et al. reported on comprehensive geriatric evaluations and effective GA-based interventions performed at the Geriatrics Service department in the Memorial Sloan Kettering Cancer Center [29]. At this center, geriatric nurse practitioners performed GAs to identify geriatric syndromes, derive patient references, and efficiently communicate with patients, caregivers, oncologists, and primary care physicians [29]. Similarly, Strohschein et al. conducted a case study of an 89-year-old man with head and neck cancer [33]. The authors concluded that oncology nurses could identify and address age-related concerns, facilitate communication, and contribute to personalized care by integrating GA tools into their practice.

In these three studies, nurses were responsible for comprehensive GAs in collaboration with a multidisciplinary team for cancer treatment [26,29,33]. Nurses conducted adequate comprehensive GAs by selecting standardized assessment tools for each domain, based on the geriatric domain framework. GAs performed by nurses led to timely interventions, proactive follow-ups, support of patient goals and values, and coordination of care. However, as GAs aim to tailor care to individual patients and improve outcomes [26], extra time must be spent on patient assessments during the decision-making process [26,33]. Thus, time is sometimes a limiting factor in the implementation of GAs.

In older people, oncology nurses can facilitate treatment planning and recovery by conducting an accurate GA. A key issue related to this is the acquisition of competencies for effectively and efficiently assessing patients in the presence of time constraints.

3.5. Provision of Available Information

Nurses play a role in the timely provision and sharing of information in the treatment decision-making process, based on a relationship of trust with the patient. A qualitative study reported that nurses attempted to compensate physicians' shortcomings by providing patients with additional information and opportunities for discussion, and sought to form trusting relationships to enable a continuity of care and facilitate access to support during treatment [21]. As older adults are sometimes reluctant to share personal information, nurses should focus on building trusting relationships with elderly patients [21]. Furthermore, pertinent patient information is not always available at the time of treatment decisions. Therefore, nurses need to continuously collect quality, available, and timely information about older adult patients, assessing what is happening in their daily lives, to enable informed treatment decisions [21].

The importance of nurses' provision of information was also indicated in studies on the perceptions of older adults with cancer. In a survey by Burton et al. of older adults with breast cancer who needed information for treatment decision-making, nearly 40% indicated that a face-to-face discussion with a nurse was their preferred source of information [22]. Furthermore, most women stated that a breast care nurse (45/55, 82%) was the ideal person with whom they would discuss their treatment decisions [22]. These results suggest the importance of the role of nurses in providing information and ensuring that women receive their preferred level and amount of information, as well as their involvement in treatment decision-making using decision support tools.

On the other hand, in a qualitative study on perceptions regarding treatment decisions in older adults with cancer, the majority of patients were satisfied with the communication with their oncologists, and none of the patients mentioned nurses as having input or providing support in their treatment decision-making process [31]. Therefore, nurses must be actively involved in decision-making processes so that their role is recognized by patients. For example, nurses may coach patients on how to seek evidence-based discussions regarding treatment options and provide supplementary education on treatment options.

McWilliams et al. conducted a qualitative study on treatment decision-making in older adults with cancer and dementia and their families, as well as HCPs, including specialized nurses [23]. One important theme was the effective communication of clinically relevant information, and the authors provided the following recommendations: taking more time with the patient, exchanging information, and understanding the options for cancer treatment. HCPs may need to speak slowly and repeat information several times to help patients and their families navigate treatment decision-making, and avoid vague descriptions of side effects, complex information, and a lack of timely information [23]. Shahrokni et.al points out that effective and efficient communication between oncologists and primary physicians or geriatricians, and nurses, especially among older people and their families, needs to be promoted to drive decision-making among older people [29].

Training in communication skills is required to promote the communication of clinically relevant information. Shen et al. evaluated a Communication Skills Training module for HCPs by applying a SDM approach to meetings with older adults with cancer and their family [32]. The results indicated a significant effect of training on overall skill; HCPs' self-efficacy in utilizing communication skills related to shared geriatric decision-making significantly increased from pre- to post-training. Communicating in a way that promotes true SDM is even more important when facing critical treatment decisions in older adults with cancer who may experience cognitive decline [32].

Studies on the perceptions of HCPs show that nurses who are trusted by patients play a role in treatment planning through the timely provision of information. Survey studies of the perceptions of older people with cancer highlighted the importance of nurses providing information, while other studies showed that there was little recognition of the input or support provided by nurses during treatment planning. Therefore, nurses need to be actively involved in the decision-making process to make patients aware of their role and to strengthen and train their communication skills.

3.6. Advocacy

Oncology nurses play an important role in advocating respect for individual values and preferences of older adults with cancer in their treatment decisions. Bridges et al. surveyed clinicians, including nurses, on the characteristics of cancer treatment decision-making in older patients with cancer and found that nurses play an important role in advocating for the patient's autonomy and the right to make informed decisions [21]. Oncology nurses involved in multidisciplinary teams focus on complex patient-centered information, such as comorbidities, psychosocial and supportive care needs, and patient preferences, indicating the importance of nurses' input in calling attention to broader issues at the meeting [21]. However, there is a difficulty in nurses providing consistent contributions to multidisciplinary team meetings [21].

On the other hand, Tariman et al. [28] reported on the preferences of older adult patients newly diagnosed with symptomatic myeloma for participation in the decision-making process and found that most patients wanted to share treatment decision-making with their physicians or make decisions themselves. Therefore, physicians and nurse practitioners must practice full disclosure of treatment options to their patients so that they can make truly informed decisions [28]. Further, the authors discussed the importance of the following roles of oncology nurses for respecting and helping individual patients with their preferences: (a) making sure patients receive disease and treatment-related information, (b) encouraging patients to express their decisional role preference to the physician, (c) developing a culture of mutual respect and value of the patient's desire for autonomy in treatment decision-making, (d) acknowledging that the patient has a right to make treatment choices, and (e) providing psychological support to the patient during decision-making, from the time of diagnosis to the end-of-life. Because the level of preference for participation is highly variable across patients, and may have personal meaning for each patient, physicians and oncology nurses must also elicit the patient's preferences, explore what participation truly means for him or her, and facilitate the patient's decision-making process [28].

The utility of decision aids (DAs) in eliciting patient preferences and providing proactive support has been evaluated. In a study of HCPs by de Angst et al. [24], 60% of nurses used DAs to elicit individual patient preferences, suggesting that DAs can be beneficial in supporting SDM. However, oncology nurses were more in favor of DAs than oncologists. In a study of older adults with advanced prostate cancer and their decision partners by Jones et al. [30], participants viewed DAs as helpful in treatment decision-making. DAs allowed issues that they were not aware of to be highlighted, thereby helping them to consider the issues in depth and discuss them with HCPs [30]. Enabling patients and decision partners to discuss issues more thoroughly and providing the time to do so improved their understanding and confidence in their decisions [30]. Additionally, DAs facilitate closer patient–HCP relationships, allowing for more patient-centered and productive conversations [30].

Older adults with cancer often have adult children or spouses involved in treatment decisions [25,27]. Therefore, nurses need to consider the impact of family involvement and family relationships on decision-making processes when supporting the patient's decision-making. Griffiths et al. indicated the necessity of an assessment that considers multiple factors and ensures psychological well-being in order to help patients apply their individualized abilities in the decision-making process [25]. Dijkman et al. explored how surgeons and nurses perceive the involvement of adult children of older patients with cancer in treatment decision-making [27]. The results indicated that nurses use the following six strategies to support positive family involvement in treatment decision-making: focus on the patient, acknowledge different perspectives, involve adult children, get to know the family system, check that the patient and family members understand the information, and stimulate communication and deliberation with adult children [27]. However, involving families in treatment decision-making also triggers specific complexities and challenges in treatment decision conversations that call for the development and implementation of practical patient- and family-centered strategies [27].

Studies on the perceptions of HCPs demonstrate the need for both nurses and physicians to fully disclose all treatment options to enable patients to make informed decisions. In particular, the preferred level of participation varies greatly from patient to patient and may have personal implications for each patient, and attention should be paid to the influence of family involvement and family relationships on decision making. Nurses need to develop communication skills to support patients' decision making, by eliciting patients' information needs and preferred level of participation.

4. Discussion

This review is unique in that it focused on the role of nurses in the treatment decisions of older adults with cancer. Previous work reported on physicians' perceptions of the decision-making process in patients with cancer [34–36] or the role of nurses [37]. One of the novel features of this review is the inclusion of data on the effect of GAs by nurses. By conducting GAs, nurses identified geriatric syndromes, elicited patient preferences, and promoted efficient communication with the patients, caregivers, and physicians. The current literature suggest that tailoring treatment decisions to a patient's frailty status and preferences leads to improvements in patient outcomes.

However, time constraints regarding the implementation of GAs were mentioned [26]. Therefore, for nurses to fulfill their expected role in a multidisciplinary team, they need to acquire competency in efficiently and effectively conducting GAs. The ability of oncology nurses to implement geriatric screening and assessment depends on additional training [33,38], as well as having the time, space, and institutional support to conduct such assessments [39,40]. Outlaw et al. provided an overview of the field of geriatric oncology and highlighted recent breakthroughs in the use of GAs in cancer care [41]. GAs are now recommended for all older adults with a new cancer diagnosis, according to recommendations from the American Society of Clinical Oncology [42], National Comprehensive Cancer Network [43], and International Society of Geriatric Oncology [44]. Further work is needed to better understand and overcome the barriers to the broad implementation and utilization of GAs [41].

Although the level of evidence was low, two case studies [29,33] provided clues regarding the development of GA training programs for nurses that are efficient and effective, as well as personalized implementation of GAs in older adults. Festen et al. showed that incorporating nurse-led GAs in decision-making may improve patient outcomes; however, future studies should use prospective cohorts in diverse cancer populations. Randomized controlled trials are needed to accumulate evidence on the effects of nurse-led GAs in decision-making [26].

Older patients with cancer are often overwhelmed by the complexity and sheer volume of information about cancer diagnosis and treatment, which hinders their access to the information they need [31,45]. The present review clarified that nurses play an important role in identifying the information needs of older patients by assessing each patient's level of understanding and helping them to understand the information. Many older patients with cancer trust their physicians and are satisfied with their provision of information; however, they also experience poor communication during the treatment decision-making process and beyond [31]. For instance, oncologists' use of medical jargon, the downplaying of treatment side effects, a lack of sensitivity, and a lack of time spent with patients are some of the issues voiced by patients in this regard [31]. Declining numeracy, lower literacy, and increasing age are associated with the desire to conserve time and energy, which may explain the strong preference for face-to-face conversations using lay language. This preference is of concern, as it may lead to inaccurate risk perceptions. Nurses need to use the teach-back method to confirm the patient's understanding of the information they receive from physicians [46], provide psychological support [37], elicit and identify individual patient-specific information needs, and facilitate accurate risk perception.

On the other hand, the present review shows that older patients with cancer sometimes do not view nurses as professionals from whom they receive important treatment-related information. Oncology nurses are key players in cancer treatment decision-making; however, they face challenges, including barriers in practice, education, institutional policies, and administration [47]. Nurses need to develop communication skills that can guide patients' information needs by employing a preemptive and proactive approach that reduces these barriers and raises nurses' roles as key persons in the care of older patients with cancer. To support the treatment and care decisions for older adults with complex health problems, physicians and nurses must have the communication skills to appropriately respond to complex patient needs through multidisciplinary-team meetings and additional information exchange as well as outside of the conference [21]. Furthermore, we believe that health care providers (HCPs) involved in the multidisciplinary-team need to share treatment and care plans using the Collaborative Care Model to facilitate smooth communication [29].

The practice of SDM is recommended as a standard approach in the decision-making process by policymakers and clinical practice guidelines [48,49]. Implementing a communication training program promotes patient engagement and SDM. The cancer treatment decision-making processes that immediately follow diagnosis occur in a team and can be characterized as medically dominated and narrowly focused on cancer pathology [21]. The importance of knowing about patients' wider health and social care needs is acknowledged by clinicians; however, they experience difficulty in ensuring that this information is available in time to inform cancer treatment decisions [21]. Thus, nurses must undertake a type of compensatory work to enable patients to engage in treatment decision-making processes and make patient-entered decisions [21]. Further, attention should shift towards exploring decision-making process modifications and providing structural support to ensure that patients with cancer with complex needs receive adequate and timely assessments and access to clinical experts with the capacity to support them in arriving at the best treatment decision [21].

DAs enable patients to fit into the treatment decision process and elicit their values and preferences, leading to proactive support by nurses [24]. A systematic review of the effectiveness of DAs for older adults showed that they improve older adults' knowledge, increase their risk perception, decrease decisional conflict, and seem to enhance participation in SDM [50]. However, few of the studies included in the present review conducted subgroup analysis in adults with low health literacy or numeracy, low-educated adults, frail patients, or other vulnerable subgroups [50]. When applying DAs to older patients with cancer, nurses need to consider several factors, including multi-morbidities, cognitive impairment, and low health literacy. In addition, more evidence concerning the effects of DAs on decision-making in older patients with cancer is needed.

Older patients with cancer often involve adult children or spouses in treatment decision-making. Family can stimulate deliberation and move the conversation beyond a mere medical perspective by considering relevant aspects of a patient's life; however, patients may withhold information in the presence of their children, or specific complexities and challenges in treatment decision conversations may be triggered [27]. Thus, nurses should develop practical strategies for triadic conversations related to treatment decision-making based on the core elements of a family system approach and family health conversations [27].

5. Limitations

One limitation of the present study is that the evidence reviewed was from a small number of studies, highlighting the need for further research that considers populations with diverse cancer types, characteristics of older adults, and diverse healthcare systems. In addition, the role of nurses may differ depending on their expertise, such as general, oncology, geriatric, and advanced practical nurses. Therefore, it is necessary to promote research that considers these subspecialties. Thematic analysis was conducted in a small number of included studies, making it difficult to extract subthemes. The present review was conducted by repeated exchanges of opinions between two researchers with different specialties (i.e., nurse and physician), from review planning to the literature searches, evaluation, and analysis. Since various professionals are involved in decision-making regarding the treatment of older people, future reviews by a multi-disciplinary expert team with collaboration among various specialties are desirable.

6. Conclusions

Cancer treatment decision-making in older patients remains a complex issue. A significant finding from the current literature is that the roles of nurses in the decision-making process of older patients with cancer involve performing an accurate GA, providing available information, and advocating respect for individual values and preferences. The role of nurses is to elicit patients' wider health and social care needs in complex decision-making processes, respecting individual references and values. However, it may be difficult for older adults and their families to perceive the complementary role of nurses in treatment decision-making, and opportunities for nurses to interact with patients may be missed due to time constraints. Further investigations focusing on the role of nurses that consider diverse cancer types, characteristics of older people, and healthcare systems are needed.

Supplementary Materials: The following supporting information can be downloaded at: https://www.mdpi.com/article/10.3390/healthcare11040546/s1, Supplementary File S1. Key words; Supplementary File S2. Searches; Supplementary File S3. Scores.

Author Contributions: Study design and concept: H.K. and Y.K.; writing the study protocol: H.K. and Y.K.; data acquisition: H.K. and Y.K.; data analysis and interpretation: H.K. and Y.K.; manuscript drafting: H.K. and Y.K.; critical revisions of the manuscript for important intellectual content: H.K. and Y.K. All authors have read and agreed to the published version of the manuscript.

Funding: This research was funded by the Japan Society for the Promotion of Science KAKENHI (Grant No.: 19H03867).

Institutional Review Board Statement: Not applicable.

Informed Consent Statement: Not applicable.

Data Availability Statement: The datasets used or analyzed during the current study available from the corresponding author on reasonable request.

Acknowledgments: This review was performed in collaboration with Ayako Tagawa and Rie Shirakura, librarians.

Conflicts of Interest: The authors declare no conflict of interest.

References

1. Pilleron, S.; Sarfati, D.; Janssen-Heijnen, M.; Vignat, J.; Ferlay, J.; Bray, F.; Soerjomataram, I. Global cancer incidence in older adults, 2012 and 2035: A population-based study. *Int. J. Cancer* **2019**, *144*, 49–58. [CrossRef]
2. Sung, H.; Ferlay, J.; Siegel, R.L.; Laversanne, M.; Soerjomataram, I.; Jemal, A.; Bray, F. Global Cancer Statistics 2020: GLOBOCAN Estimates of Incidence and Mortality Worldwide for 36 Cancers in 185 Countries. *CA Cancer J. Clin.* **2021**, *71*, 209–249. [CrossRef]
3. Balducci, L. Management of cancer in the elderly. *Oncology* **2006**, *20*, 135–143.
4. Handforth, C.; Burkinshaw, R.; Freeman, J.; Brown, J.E.; Snowden, J.A.; Coleman, R.E.; Greenfield, D.M. Comprehensive geriatric assessment and decision-making in older men with incurable but manageable (chronic) cancer. *Support. Care Cancer* **2019**, *27*, 1755–1763. [CrossRef]
5. Rostoft, S.; O'Donovan, A.; Soubeyran, P.; Alibhai, S.M.H.; Hamaker, M.E. Geriatric Assessment and Management in Cancer. *J. Clin. Oncol.* **2021**, *39*, 2058–2067. [CrossRef]
6. Wan-Chow-Wah, D.; Monette, J.; Monette, M.; Sourial, N.; Retornaz, F.; Batist, G.; Puts, M.T.; Bergman, H. Difficulties in decision making regarding chemotherapy for older cancer patients: A census of cancer physicians. *Crit. Rev. Oncol.* **2011**, *78*, 45–58. [CrossRef]
7. Soto-Perez-De-Celis, E.; Li, D.; Yuan, Y.; Lau, Y.M.; Hurria, A. Functional versus chronological age: Geriatric assessments to guide decision making in older patients with cancer. *Lancet Oncol.* **2018**, *19*, e305–e316. [CrossRef]
8. van der Poel, M.W.; Mulder, W.J.; Ossenkoppele, G.J.; Maartense, E.; Wijermans, P.; Hoogendoorn, M.; Schouten, H.C. Comorbidity and treatment decision-making in elderly non-Hodgkin's lymphoma patients: A survey among haematologists. *Neth. J. Med.* **2014**, *72*, 165–169.
9. Hamaker, M.E.; Molder, M.T.; Thielen, N.; van Munster, B.C.; Schiphorst, A.H.; van Huis, L.H. The effect of a geriatric evaluation on treatment decisions and outcome for older cancer patients–A systematic review. *J. Geriatr. Oncol.* **2018**, *9*, 430–440. [CrossRef]
10. Shin, D.W.; Cho, J.; Roter, D.L.; Kim, S.Y.; Park, J.H.; Yang, H.K.; Lee, H.W.; Kweon, S.-S.; Kang, Y.S.; Park, K. Patient's Cognitive Function and Attitudes towards Family Involvement in Cancer Treatment Decision Making: A Patient-Family Caregiver Dyadic Analysis. *Cancer Res. Treat.* **2018**, *50*, 681–690. [CrossRef]
11. Kadambi, S.; Loh, K.P.; Dunne, R.; Magnuson, A.; Maggiore, R.; Zittel, J.; Flannery, M.; Inglis, J.; Gilmore, N.; Mohamed, M.; et al. Older adults with cancer and their caregivers—current landscape and future directions for clinical care. *Nat. Rev. Clin. Oncol.* **2020**, *17*, 742–755. [CrossRef] [PubMed]

12. Mohile, S.G.; Dale, W.; Somerfield, M.R.; Schonberg, M.A.; Boyd, C.M.; Burhenn, P.; Canin, B.; Cohen, H.J.; Holmes, H.M.; Hopkins, J.O.; et al. Practical Assessment and Management of Vulnerabilities in Older Patients Receiving Chemotherapy: ASCO Guideline for Geriatric Oncology. *J. Clin. Oncol.* **2018**, *36*, 2326–2347. [CrossRef]
13. Hurria, A.; Mohile, S.; Gajra, A.; Klepin, H.; Muss, H.; Chapman, A.; Feng, T.; Smith, D.; Sun, C.-L.; De Glas, N.; et al. Validation of a Prediction Tool for Chemotherapy Toxicity in Older Adults With Cancer. *J. Clin. Oncol.* **2016**, *34*, 2366–2371. [CrossRef] [PubMed]
14. Mohile, S.G.; Velarde, C.; Hurria, A.; Magnuson, A.; Lowenstein, L.; Pandya, C.; O'Donovan, A.; Gorawara-Bhat, R.; Dale, W. Geriatric Assessment-Guided Care Processes for Older Adults: A Delphi Consensus of Geriatric Oncology Experts. *J. Natl. Compr. Cancer Netw.* **2015**, *13*, 1120–1130. [CrossRef]
15. Kane, H.L.; Halpern, M.T.; Squiers, L.B.; Treiman, K.A.; McCormack, L.A. Implementing and evaluating shared decision making in oncology practice. *CA A Cancer J. Clin.* **2014**, *64*, 377–388. [CrossRef] [PubMed]
16. Volker, D.L.; Kahn, D.; Penticuff, J.H. Patient Control and End-of-Life Care Part I: The Advanced Practice Nurse Perspective. *Oncol. Nurs. Forum* **2004**, *31*, 945–953. [CrossRef] [PubMed]
17. Tariman, J.D.; Mehmeti, E.; Spawn, N.; McCarter, S.P.; Bishop-Royse, J.; Garcia, I.; Hartle, L.; Szubski, K. Oncology Nursing and Shared Decision Making for Cancer Treatment. *Clin. J. Oncol. Nurs.* **2016**, *20*, 560–563. [CrossRef] [PubMed]
18. Page, M.J.; McKenzie, J.E.; Bossuyt, P.M.; Boutron, I.; Hoffmann, T.C.; Mulrow, C.D.; Shamseer, L.; Tetzlaff, J.M.; Akl, E.A.; Brennan, S.E.; et al. The PRISMA 2020 Statement: An Updated Guideline for Reporting Systematic Reviews. *BMJ* **2021**, *372*, n71. [CrossRef] [PubMed]
19. Hong, Q.N.; Pluye, P.; Fabregues, S.; Bartlett, G.; Boardman, F.; Cargo, M.; Dagenais, P.; Gagnon, M.-P.; Griffiths, F.; Nicolau, B.; et al. Mixed Methods Appraisal Tool (MMAT), Version Registration of Copyright. 2018, p. 1148552. Available online: http://mixedmethodsappraisaltoolpublic.pbworks.com/ (accessed on 15 September 2022).
20. Thomas, J.; Harden, A. Methods for the thematic synthesis of qualitative research in systematic reviews. *BMC Med. Res. Methodol.* **2008**, *8*, 45. [CrossRef] [PubMed]
21. Bridges, J.; Hughes, J.; Farrington, N.; Richardson, A. Cancer treatment decision-making processes for older patients with complex needs: A qualitative study. *BMJ Open* **2015**, *5*, e009674. [CrossRef]
22. Burton, M.; Kilner, K.; Wyld, L.; Lifford, K.J.; Gordon, F.; Allison, A.; Reed, M.; Collins, K.A. Information needs and decision-making preferences of older women offered a choice between surgery and primary endocrine therapy for early breast cancer. *Psycho-Oncology* **2017**, *26*, 2094–2100. [CrossRef]
23. McWilliams, L.; Farrell, C.; Keady, J.; Swarbrick, C.; Burgess, L.; Grande, G.; Bellhouse, S.; Yorke, J. Cancer-related information needs and treatment decision-making experiences of people with dementia in England: A multiple perspective qualitative study. *BMJ Open* **2018**, *8*, e020250. [CrossRef]
24. de Angst, I.B.; Kil, P.J.; Bangma, C.H.; Takkenberg, J.J. Should we involve patients more actively? Perspectives of the multidisciplinary team on shared decision-making for older patients with metastatic castration-resistant prostate cancer. *J. Geriatr. Oncol.* **2019**, *10*, 653–658. [CrossRef]
25. Griffiths, A.W.; Ashley, L.; Kelley, R.; Cowdell, F.; Collinson, M.; Mason, E.; Farrin, A.; Henry, A.; Inman, H.; Surr, C. Decision-making in cancer care for people living with dementia. *Psycho-Oncology* **2020**, *29*, 1347–1354. [CrossRef]
26. Festen, S.; van der Wal-Huisman, H.; van der Leest, A.H.; Reyners, A.K.; de Bock, G.H.; de Graeff, P.; van Leeuwen, B.L. The effect of treatment modifications by an onco-geriatric MDT on one-year mortality, days spent at home and postoperative complications. *J. Geriatr. Oncol.* **2021**, *12*, 779–785. [CrossRef]
27. Dijkman, B.L.; Paans, W.; Van der Wal-Huisman, H.; van Leeuwen, B.L.; Luttik, M.L. Involvement of adult children in treatment decision-making for older patients with cancer—a qualitative study of perceptions and experiences of oncology surgeons and nurses. *Support. Care Cancer* **2022**, *30*, 9203–9210. [CrossRef]
28. Tariman, J.D.; Doorenbos, A.; Schepp, K.G.; Becker, P.S.; Berry, D.L. Patient, physician and contextual factors are influential in the treatment decision making of older adults newly diagnosed with symptomatic myeloma. *Cancer Treat. Commun.* **2014**, *2*, 34–47. [CrossRef]
29. Shahrokni, A.; Kim, S.J.; Bosl, G.J.; Korc-Grodzicki, B. How We Care for an Older Patient With Cancer. *J. Oncol. Pract.* **2017**, *13*, 95–102. [CrossRef]
30. Jones, R.A.; Hollen, P.J.; Wenzel, J.; Weiss, G.; Song, D.; Sims, T.; Petroni, G. Understanding Advanced Prostate Cancer Decision Making Utilizing an Interactive Decision Aid. *Cancer Nurs.* **2018**, *41*, 2–10. [CrossRef] [PubMed]
31. Sattar, S.; Alibhai, S.M.; Fitch, M.; Krzyzanowska, M.; Leighl, N.; Puts, M.T. Chemotherapy and radiation treatment decision-making experiences of older adults with cancer: A qualitative study. *J. Geriatr. Oncol.* **2018**, *9*, 47–52. [CrossRef]
32. Shen, M.J.; Manna, R.; Banerjee, S.C.; Nelson, C.J.; Alexander, K.; Alici, Y.; Gangai, N.; Parker, P.A.; Korc-Grodzicki, B. Incorporating shared decision making into communication with older adults with cancer and their caregivers: Development and evaluation of a geriatric shared decision-making communication skills training module. *Patient Educ. Couns.* **2020**, *103*, 2328–2334. [CrossRef] [PubMed]
33. Strohschein, F.J.; Loucks, A.; Jin, R.; Vanderbyl, B. Comprehensive Geriatric Assessment: A Case Report on Personalizing Cancer Care of an Older Adult Patient With Head and Neck Cancer. *Clin. J. Oncol. Nurs.* **2020**, *24*, 514–525. [CrossRef] [PubMed]
34. Hanna, S.A.; Marta, G.N.; Santos, F.S. The physician and updates in cancer treatment: When to stop? *Rev. Assoc. Med. Bras.* **2011**, *57*, 588–593. [CrossRef] [PubMed]

35. Tariman, J.D.; Berry, D.L.; Cochrane, B.; Doorenbos, A.; Schepp, K.G. Physician, Patient, and Contextual Factors Affecting Treatment Decisions in Older Adults with Cancer and Models of Decision Making: A Literature Review. *Oncol. Nurs. Forum* 2012, *39*, E70–E83. [CrossRef]
36. Broc, G.; Gana, K.; Denost, Q.; Quintard, B. Decision-making in rectal and colorectal cancer: Systematic review and qualitative analysis of surgeons' preferences. *Psychol. Health Med.* 2017, *22*, 434–448. [CrossRef]
37. Tariman, J.; Szubski, K. The Evolving Role of the Nurse During the Cancer Treatment Decision-Making Process: A Literature Review. *Clin. J. Oncol. Nurs.* 2015, *19*, 548–556. [CrossRef] [PubMed]
38. Nightingale, G.; Burhenn, P.S.; Puts, M.; Stolz-Baskett, P.; Haase, K.R.; Sattar, S.; Kenis, C. Integrating Nurses and Allied Health Professionals in the care of older adults with cancer: A report from the International Society of Geriatric Oncology Nursing and Allied Health Interest Group. *J. Geriatr. Oncol.* 2020, *11*, 187–190. [CrossRef]
39. Strohschein, F.; Haase, K.; Puts, M.; Jin, R.; Newton, L.; Fitch, M.; Loucks, A.; Kenis, C. Facilitating a Canadian conversation about oncology nurses' role in optimizing care of older adults with cancer: Preliminary insights. *J. Geriatr. Oncol.* 2019, *10* (Suppl. 1), S84. [CrossRef]
40. Strohschein, F.J.; Newton, L.; Puts, M.; Jin, R.; Haase, K.; Plante, A.; Loucks, A.; Kenis, C.; Fitch, M. Optimizing the Care of Older Canadians with Cancer and their Families: A Statement Articulating the Position and Contribution of Canadian Oncology Nurses. *Can. Oncol. Nurs. J.* 2021, *31*, 352–356. [PubMed]
41. Outlaw, D.; Abdallah, M.; A Gil-Jr, L.; Giri, S.; Hsu, T.; Krok-Schoen, J.L.; Liposits, G.; Madureira, T.; Marinho, J.; Subbiah, I.M.; et al. The Evolution of Geriatric Oncology and Geriatric Assessment over the Past Decade. *Semin. Radiat. Oncol.* 2022, *32*, 98–108. [CrossRef]
42. Giri, S.; Chakiba, C.; Shih, Y.Y.; Chan, W.L.; Krok-Schoen, J.L.; Presley, C.J.; Williams, G.R.; Subbiah, I.M. Integration of geriatric assessment into routine oncologic care and advances in geriatric oncology: A young International Society of Geriatric Oncology Report of the 2020 American Society of Clinical Oncology (ASCO) annual meeting. *J. Geriatr. Oncol.* 2020, *11*, 1324–1328. [CrossRef]
43. DuMontier, C.; Sedrak, M.S.; Soo, W.K.; Kenis, C.; Williams, G.R.; Haase, K.; Harneshaug, M.; Mian, H.; Loh, K.P.; Rostoft, S.; et al. Arti Hurria and the progress in integrating the geriatric assessment into oncology: Young International Society of Geriatric Oncology review paper. *J. Geriatr. Oncol.* 2020, *11*, 203–211. [CrossRef] [PubMed]
44. Extermann, M.; Brain, E.; Canin, B.; Cherian, M.N.; Cheung, K.L.; de Glas, N.; Devi, B.; Hamaker, M.; Kanesvaran, R.; Karnakis, T.; et al. Priorities for the global advancement of care for older adults with cancer: An update of the International Society of Geriatric Oncology Priorities Initiative. *Lancet Oncol.* 2021, *22*, e29–e36. [CrossRef] [PubMed]
45. Chouliara, Z.; Kearney, N.; Stott, D.; Molassiotis, A.; Miller, M. Perceptions of older people with cancer of information, decision making and treatment: A systematic review of selected literature. *Ann. Oncol.* 2004, *15*, 1596–1602. [CrossRef] [PubMed]
46. Choi, S.; Choi, J. Effects of the teach-back method among cancer patients: A systematic review of the literature. *Support. Care Cancer* 2021, *29*, 7259–7268. [CrossRef]
47. McCarter, S.P.; Tariman, J.D.; Spawn, N.; Mehmeti, E.; Bishop-Royse, J.; Garcia, I.; Hartle, L.; Szubski, K. Barriers and Promoters to Participation in the Era of Shared Treatment Decision-Making. *West. J. Nurs. Res.* 2016, *38*, 1282–1297. [CrossRef]
48. Carmona, C.; Crutwell, J.; Burnham, M.; Polak, L.; Guideline Committee. Shared decision-making: Summary of NICE guidance. *BMJ* 2021, *373*, n1430. [CrossRef]
49. Maes-Carballo, M.; Muñoz-Núñez, I.; Martín-Díaz, M.; Mignini, L.; Bueno-Cavanillas, A.; Khan, K.S. Shared decision making in breast cancer treatment guidelines: Development of a quality assessment tool and a systematic review. *Health Expect.* 2020, *23*, 1045–1064. [CrossRef]
50. van Weert, J.C.; Bolle, S.; van Dulmen, S.; Jansen, J. Older cancer patients' information and communication needs: What they want is what they get? *Patient Educ. Couns.* 2013, *92*, 388–397. [CrossRef]

Disclaimer/Publisher's Note: The statements, opinions and data contained in all publications are solely those of the individual author(s) and contributor(s) and not of MDPI and/or the editor(s). MDPI and/or the editor(s) disclaim responsibility for any injury to people or property resulting from any ideas, methods, instructions or products referred to in the content.

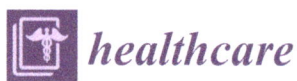

Article

The Effect of a Nurse-Led Family Involvement Program on Anxiety and Depression in Patients with Advanced-Stage Hepatocellular Carcinoma

Sukhuma Klankaew [1], Suthisa Temthup [1,*], Kittikorn Nilmanat [2] and Margaret I. Fitch [3]

[1] Songklanagarind Hospital, Faculty of Medicine, Prince of Songkla University, Songkhla 90110, Thailand
[2] Faculty of Nursing, Prince of Songkla University, Songkhla 90110, Thailand
[3] Bloomberg Faculty of Nursing, University of Toronto, Toronto, ON M4C 4V9, Canada
* Correspondence: tsutisa@medicine.psu.ac.th

Abstract: Psychological distress is commonly reported in patients with advanced cancer. Family is considered a psychological supporter for patients during their cancer journey. This study aimed to examine the effect of a nurse-led family involvement program on anxiety and depression in patients with advanced hepatocellular cancer. This is a quasi-experimental study with a two-group, pre–post-test design. Forty-eight participants were recruited at a male medical ward in a university hospital in Southern Thailand, and assigned to either the experimental or the control group. The experimental group received the nurse-led family involvement program, while the control group received only conventional care. Instruments included a demographic data form, clinical data form, and the Hospital Anxiety and Depression Scale. Data analyses were performed using descriptive statistics, chi-square, Fisher's exact test, and *t*-test. The results revealed that the mean scores of anxiety and depression in the experimental group at post-test were significantly lower than on the pretest and significantly lower than those of the control group. The results indicate that a nurse-led family involvement program has a short-term effect on the reduction of anxiety and depression in male patients with advanced HCC. The program can be useful for nurses to encourage family caregivers to engage in patient care during hospitalization.

Keywords: anxiety; depression; family involvement; hepatocellular carcinoma; palliative care

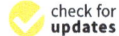

Citation: Klankaew, S.; Temthup, S.; Nilmanat, K.; Fitch, M.I. The Effect of a Nurse-Led Family Involvement Program on Anxiety and Depression in Patients with Advanced-Stage Hepatocellular Carcinoma. *Healthcare* 2023, 11, 460. https://doi.org/10.3390/healthcare11040460

Academic Editor: Daniele Giansanti

Received: 24 December 2022
Revised: 2 February 2023
Accepted: 3 February 2023
Published: 5 February 2023

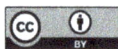

Copyright: © 2023 by the authors. Licensee MDPI, Basel, Switzerland. This article is an open access article distributed under the terms and conditions of the Creative Commons Attribution (CC BY) license (https://creativecommons.org/licenses/by/4.0/).

1. Introduction

Hepatocellular cancer (HCC) is a common cancer, in which most patients have a poor prognosis [1]. The disease is typically discovered late in the course of the illness, as it is challenging to identify in the early stages [2]. It was reported that between 15–20% of patients with HCC arrive at the doctor's office when they are in an advanced disease stage and are apt to have a survival time of only 3–4 months after diagnosis [3]. Of these patients with advanced HCC, 94% die while in hospital [4]. Due to poor prognosis, major hepatology societies recommend integrating early supportive and palliative care for patients with HCC [1].

Psychosocial consequences are commonly reported among persons with cancer, although individuals may experience depression and anxiety differently, as a result of personal, psychological, social, and environmental factors as well as the type of cancer and medical treatments [5]. Anxiety and depression are reflective conditions regarding adaptation to the illness and may indicate the patient is having difficulty coping effectively with stress. Patients with advanced HCC have significant psychological distress [4]. A recent systematic review reported that 40% of patients with metastatic HCC have anxiety and depression [6] with HCC progression associated with depression [7]. Several other factors are related to anxiety and depression in patients with HCC, including female gender, higher Charlson comorbidity index scores, and liver cirrhosis [6]. In addition, advanced Barcelona

Clinic Liver Cancer (BCLC) stage and undergoing liver resection are significantly related to more severe physical and psychological symptoms in these patients [2]. A systematic review focusing on factors associated with heightened risk for depression in cancer patients found that patients without personal relationships were up to four times more likely to experience depression compared with patients who were in relationships [8].

Furthermore, a recent systematic scoping review reported in patients with advanced cancer that higher levels of distress, depression, and anxiety were linked to higher levels of unmet need demands in the major domains (e.g., physical, emotional, practical) and across the broad spectrum of cancer types [9]. Wang et al. [10] examined unmet care needs of advanced cancer patients. Unmet psychological and physical needs were identified as two areas of focus for patients with advanced cancer, while family and friends' support was the most common unmet social need.

In Thailand, nearly 40% of patients with HCC who come to see a doctor have already entered an advanced stage of disease [11,12]. These patients are often hospitalized and receive palliative care to relieve distressful symptoms. However, being hospitalized may result in experiencing a sense of loneliness and social isolation. Riedl and Schüßler [8] reported that depression and emotional distress were consistently related to social deprivation and poor social support. Recently, Temtap and Nilmanat [13] found that hospitalized patients with advanced HCC experienced high levels of anxiety and depression.

In addressing the need for psychological care for cancer patients, Weis [14] suggested a stepped-care approach, including systematic need assessment, integrated psychosocial care delivery by care managers that range from counseling to individual psychotherapy, and appropriate professional supervision. A randomized control trial of a comprehensive education and care program was found to be beneficial in reducing anxiety and depression in patients with hepatocellular carcinoma who underwent surgery [15]. In addition, a recent systematic review reported beneficial effects of psycho-oncological intervention on the reduction of anxiety and depression symptoms for this population [6].

Family support is a common form of social support and has been reported to enhance effective coping strategies [16,17] and reduce anxiety among patients with cancer [18]. Family members may be in the best position to provide emotional support to these patients during their cancer journey. It is suggested that people living with cancer may benefit from psychosocial interventions that are focused on patient and family caregivers [19]. However, at present, family involvement in an acute care hospital setting is characterized by poor communication, a lack of agreement of caregiving roles, and a lack of cooperation and collaboration between family caregivers and nurses [20]. Culture also influences the level of family involvement in treatment decision making, especially for older adults with cancer [21].

To date, several psychological interventions have been conducted in patients with some cancer types, such as prostate cancer [22,23] and breast cancer [24,25]. However, there is a paucity of literature on family involvement interventions that focus on psychosocial aspects, particularly in adult acute care hospital settings. Thailand is a family-oriented society, and family caregivers are often present in healthcare facilities during a patient's hospitalization. Frequently, family members are used for inpatient care. To our knowledge, no other intervention study has provided a family engagement program to reduce psychological distress among Thai patients with HCC. We anticipated that an intervention program to promote family involvement could fulfill the care need, consequently alleviating anxiety and depression in patients with advanced cancer.

Conceptual Framework and Literature Review

This study used the family support concept [26] and the literature review on the needs of patients with HCC, as well as the roles of nurses in palliative care [17,27–30] to develop an intervention program, namely the nurse-led family involvement program. Furthermore, the family involvement program was designed and centered on facilitating communication within the family. Previous studies found that a communication-focused approach enhanced the quality of life and coping skills of family caregivers for patients with cancer [27].

People with advanced HCC experience physical symptoms as well as difficulty performing daily tasks. They, therefore, have a need for assistance. Hien, Chanruangvanich, and Thosingha [31] examined palliative care needs among patients with HCC. They found that patients who have high levels of physical symptoms, anxiety, and depression but low social support would have high palliative care needs [31]. Palliative care support for patients with HCC includes symptom management, decisional support, care coordination, and psychosocial support [1,32]. Nurses can provide palliative care to patients with HCC and their families at any stage of the disease.

In order to respond to the palliative care needs of patients with HCC holistically, we consider families as the main source of support for patients with HCC. Family support can be given in the form of information, emotional support, and practical assistance to sick persons [26]. Therefore, our program involved family members of patients with HCC to engage in four domains of care activities, including information sharing, care decisions, care provision, and psychological support. Nurses facilitate family involvement during visiting time. It was recommended that healthcare providers must acknowledge the presence of the family and routinely interact with them [28]. Information sharing is one of the education sessions. Nurses provide health education tailored to patients' information needs. Evidence reveals that patients may feel difficulty comprehending disease-specific information provided by medical doctors [33]. Family members help patients in remembering or recalling information, giving information directly to the doctor, or clarifying instructions from the doctor so the patient can understand and seek necessary information [34]. The program facilitates patients and family caregivers to interact with the nurse and ask questions. Furthermore, a previous systematic study found that fatigue was reported as the most prominent physical unmet need among patients with advanced cancer [10]. Fatigue was a common physical health problem experienced by patients with HCC [35,36]. Nurses involve families to provide bedside care for patients with HCC.

Effective communication and shared decision making were reported as one of the most important elements in end-of-life care [29]. Similar to many Asian patients, Thai families played a crucial role in treatment decisions. These patients preferred to share decisions about cancer treatments with their family [30]. A previous study found that making decisions alone was linked to lower emotional, social, and spiritual wellbeing among Asian patients with advanced cancer, whereas making decisions jointly with doctors and family was linked to greater social and spiritual wellbeing [37]. Spending more time discussing treatment choices with family members helps patients cope with their cancer diagnosis and promotes cognitive processing, both of which may eventually reduce the patient's stress levels [38]. Psychological support is another aspect of the program. Nurses encourage the family to provide emotional and psychological support to their loved ones. It was found previously that during cancer treatment, patients frequently did not want to express difficult feelings with nurses [39]. Patients may be more willing to share their concerns with their family members. Support, particularly emotional support, from family members is crucial for coping with cancer [17]. They believed that their families were crucial in helping them cope with their condition and face the doubts and anxieties that came with receiving a cancer diagnosis [40].

From a literature review, the family support and palliative care concept seems to be appropriate for guiding an intervention to reduce anxiety and depression in patients with advanced-stage HCC. Therefore, we were interested in examining the effect of a nurse-led family involvement program to reduce anxiety and depression of patients with advanced HCC.

2. Materials and Methods

2.1. Design

This study used a quasi-experimental study with a two-group, pre–post-test design. The purpose of this study was to compare anxiety and depression between the experimental group who received a nurse-led family involvement program and the control group who received only conventional care. This report follows Transparent Reporting of Evaluations with Non-randomized Designs (TREND) [41].

2.2. Participants

The authors recruited persons with HCC who met the inclusion criteria at a male medical unit in a university hospital in Southern Thailand. The inclusion criteria for persons with cancer were (1) knowing their diagnosis of advanced hepatocellular cancer according to the Diagnostic Statistical Manual-IV diagnostic criteria (BCLC stage C) or (BCLC stage D) and receiving palliative care treatments, (2) being fully conscious and able to communicate in Thai, and (3) having a primary family caregiver to provide care continuously in the hospital. The exclusion criteria were (1) being critically ill and experiencing severely acute exacerbations such as difficulty breathing or acute renal failure, (2) declining to participate in the study, and (3) having an anxiety or depression score higher than 11 on the Thai version of Hospital Anxiety and Depression Scale (HADs-Thai version) [42].

The sample size was calculated using Polit and Beck's [43] recommendation that the minimum sample size for a quasi-experimental study was 20–30 subjects. In this study, the sample size was determined as 20 per group, with an additional 20% in each group to account for any dropout of subjects. A total of 48 eligible patients were recruited (24 subjects per group) by the researcher and allocated to the experimental or control groups using a simple random allocation method. During the study, 8 subjects were excluded and withdrawn from the study due to high psychological distress (3) and severity of disease (5), respectively, leaving 20 subjects per group.

For each patient, a family member was also recruited. The inclusion criteria for the family members were (1) being a primary caregiver who provides care continuously for the patient during the cancer treatment process in the hospital, (2) being aware of the advanced stage of cancer of the patient, (3) being 18 years and older, (4) being willing to participate in the study and able to attend all sessions of the four-day intervention program (for experimental group), and (5) being able to read and understand the Thai language.

2.3. Interventions

All patient participants received conventional nursing care according to the clinical practice and palliative care guidelines in our Palliative Care Manual of the Nursing Service Department. The conventional care included routine monitoring of vital signs and hemorrhage signs; routine blood and urine laboratory examinations; management of discomfort symptoms, diet, activity, personal hygiene care, and so on.

The nurse-led family involvement program was developed by the research team based on a literature review regarding the needs of patients with advanced cancer and the concept of family support and palliative care [17,26–30]. The program contents and activities were reviewed and validated by three experts and revised as recommended before implementation. The nurse-led family involvement program intervention focused on four aspects of family involvement, including information sharing, care decisions, care provision, and psychological support. Both the patient and family member received the intervention together on the first day of hospitalization and continued for four days in a row. Each session was held at the patient's bedside and took between 30–60 min during family visiting time. A member of the research team provided the intervention. In addition, a caregiver booklet on caring for patients with advanced HCC was provided. The content of the booklet included the caregivers' role in supportive caring activities, self-care activities, symptoms, and symptom management in HCC. The details of the program are presented in Table 1.

Table 1. Schedule and contents for the 4-day nurse-led family involvement program.

Day	Duration (Minutes)	Key Aspects of Involvement	Activities
1	15–20	Pretest	- Collecting HADs questionnaire from patients by RAs
	30–40	- Information sharing - Care provision - Psychological care	- Establishing relationship and building trust with the patient and their family caregiver - Encouraging them to share experiences and to express feelings and thoughts related to illness and care needs - Addressing the significant roles of family caregivers along the cancer journey - Providing information about the disease, treatment plans, and care demands of patients to the patient and their family caregivers - Providing family caregivers a booklet on caring for patients with advance HCC - Encouraging family caregivers to engage in care provision of the patients, including personal hygiene care, comfort care
2–4	40–60	- Information sharing - Care decisions - Care provision - Psychological care	- Involving family caregivers during providing health information to the patients and encouraging them to ask questions if there are any - Explaining about patients' symptoms, treatment, and care plan, and encouraging family caregivers to review about patient's problems - Involving family caregivers in conversations with the physicians - Facilitating open discussion among family and listening attentively - Consulting the family physician to initiate a family meeting and share any decisions - Encouraging family caregivers to be involved in care provision for the patients such as bed baths, comfort care - Providing information related to psychological care activities to family caregivers, such as listening, use of touch, being present, using positive words, or relaxation techniques
5	15–20	Post-test	- Collecting HADs questionnaire from patients by Ras

2.4. Instruments

The instruments utilized to gather data on demographic characteristics of patients and family caregivers as well as clinical data were developed by the PI for the purposes of the study. The items collected data on (1) patient characteristics, including age, religious affiliation, educational level, marital status, occupation, sufficiency of income to cover current expenses, and types of health insurance; (2) family caregivers' characteristics, including gender, age, educational level, occupation, and relationship with patient; and (3) patient clinical data, including Thai Palliative Performance Scale score [44], the severity of the disease with Child Pugh score [45], and times since diagnosis.

The instrument used to collect anxiety and depression data was the Hospital Anxiety and Depression Scale (HADS), developed by Zigmond and Snaith [46]. This self-rating scale has two subscales: one measures depression with seven items and the other measures anxiety with seven items. Each item is scored on a 4-point (0–3) Likert scale and rates how the individual has been feeling in the past week. The scores of 0–7 indicate "normal", while 8–10, 11–14, and 15–21, "indicate mild", "moderate", and "severe", respectively. In this study, the Thai version of HADs was used [42], and the Cronbach's alpha coefficient was found to be 0.89 for the anxiety subscale and 0.82 for the depression subscale.

2.5. Ethical Considerations

The study was conducted in accordance with the Declaration of Helsinki and was approved by the Institutional Review Board of the Faculty of Medicine, Prince of Songkla University (EC 62-131-15-7). All eligible subjects were informed of the objectives and processes of the study, the benefits and potential risks, time required, rights to privacy, confidentiality, and ability to withdraw without losing healthcare service benefits. They were given opportunities to ask questions. All subjects signed consent forms before the study participation. Furthermore, written informed consent has been obtained from the patients to publish this paper.

2.6. Data Collection and Intervention

After IRB approval, ward nurses informed the research team about new admission of patients with HCC. A member of the research team (ST) then recruited patients who met the inclusion criteria and agreed to participate in the study. She subsequently introduced herself to the patients' family caregivers and invited them to participate in the study. Participants in both groups were informed about the study before signing the informed consent form.

After consent was obtained, patients and family caregivers were asked to complete the demographic data. The experimental group then received the family involvement program and conventional care. The PI (SK) provided the intervention to the experimental group. The control group received conventional care.

Two research assistants (RA) who were nurses from the internal medicine ward and trained for data collection and research ethics collected the data. The RA completed the clinical data form and HAD questionnaires in both patient groups at the pretest on the first day of hospitalization and post-test on the fifth day of hospitalization. RAs were unaware of the group assignment.

Of the 48 patients with advanced HCC assessed for eligibility, all were invited to participate in the study. However, only 23 patients in the experimental group and 22 patients in the control group met the inclusion criteria. During the study, three participants in the experimental group and two in the control group withdrew because of progression in severity of disease. A total of 40 participants completed the study, with 20 in the experimental group and 20 in the control group (Figure 1). Data were collected from July 2019 to August 2021.

2.7. Data Analysis

Data were analyzed using R program. Descriptive analysis was performed for all variables and presented as mean and standard deviation, count (percentage), or median and interquartile range. To compare differences between the two groups at baseline, chi-square statistical analyses and Fisher's exact test were employed. Comparison between groups was determined by paired t-test, independent-sample t-test, Chi-square test, or Wilcoxon rank sum test depending on the type of data.

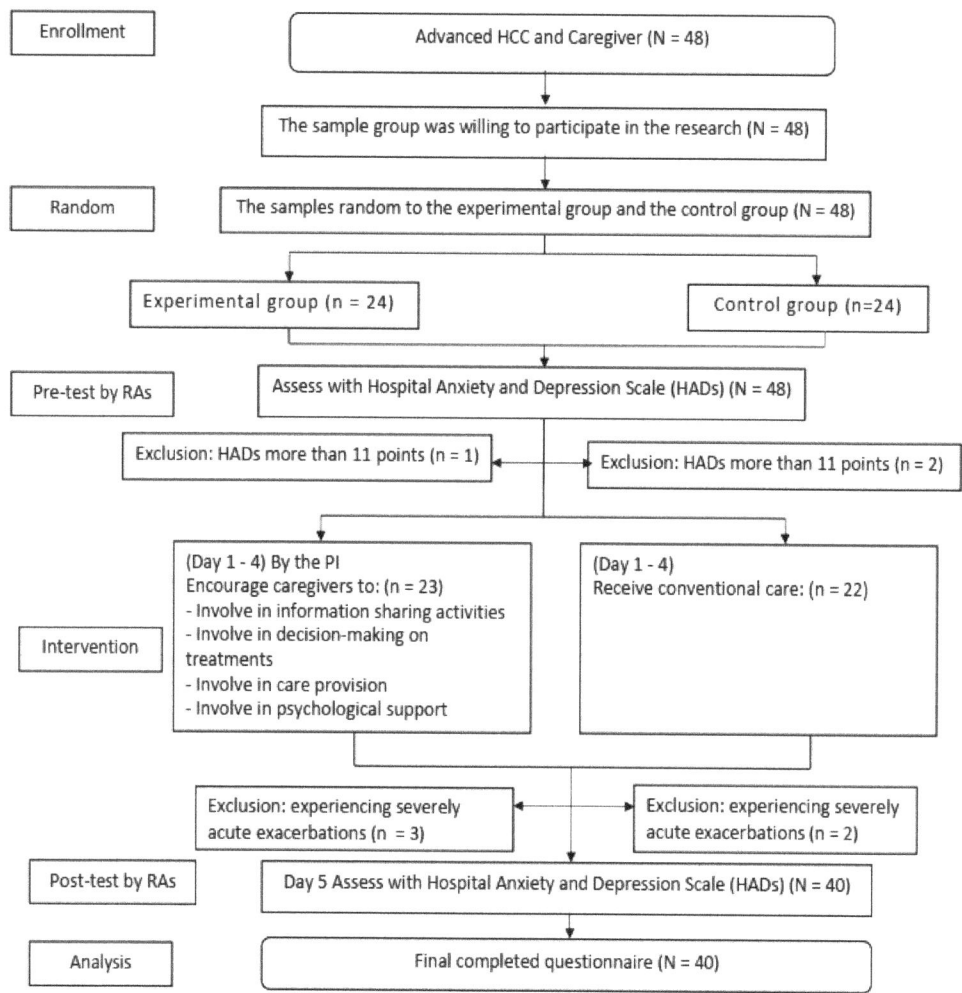

Figure 1. Flow diagram of the participants in the study.

3. Results

Forty participants completed the study. Twenty participants were in both the experimental and control groups. Demographics regarding age, marital status, educational level, occupation, age of caregivers, relationship with caregiver did not differ statistically between experimental and control groups. For clinical data, PPS scores, Child Pugh scores, and time since diagnosis were not significantly different between the two groups (Table 2).

The means and standard deviations for anxiety and depression in both groups at baseline are presented in Table 3. The independent *t*-test was used to compare the scores of two outcome variable measures at baseline. There were no significant differences in the overall mean scores for anxiety and depression between experimental and control groups.

Table 2. Basic characteristics of patients with HCC in the experimental and control groups (N = 40).

Characteristics	Group		Statistic Results	p-Value
	Intervention (20) n(%)	Control (20) n(%)		
Religious affiliation [#]			0.404	0.525
Buddhism	10 (50)	12 (60)		
Islam	10 (50)	8 (40)		
Educational level [#]			0.150	0.928
Primary school	6 (30)	5 (25)		
Secondary school/high school/diploma	8 (40)	9 (45)		
Bachelor degree/or higher	6 (30)	6 (30)		
Marital status [##]			1.619	0.695
Single	1 (5)	1 (5)		
Married	17 (85)	14 (70)		
Widowed/divorced/separated	2 (10)	5 (25)		
Occupation [##]			0.648	0.878
Unemployed	15 (75)	13 (65)		
Government officer	3 (15)	5 (25)		
Merchant	2 (10)	2 (10)		
Caregivers' age (years) [#]			0.784	0.661
<60	16 (80)	18 (90)		
≥60	4 (20)	2 (10)		
Relationship with patients [#]			0.114	0.736
Spouse	14 (70)	13 (65)		
Daughter/son	6 (30)	7 (35)		
Caregivers' gender [##]			0.173	0.500
Female	16 (80)	17 (85)		
Male	4 (20)	3 (15)		
Caregivers' occupation [#]			3.552	0.314
Farmer/gardener	9 (45)	12 (60)		
Merchant	9 (45)	4 (20)		
Government officer	2 (10)	3 (15)		
Unemployed	0	1 (5)		
PPS [##]			1.726	1.000
End-of-life phase	0 (0)	1 (5)		
Transition phase	18 (90)	18 (90)		
Stable phase	2 (10)	1 (5)		
Severity of disease (Child Pugh score) [#]			0.100	0.752
Child Pugh score B	11 (55)	10 (50)		
Child Pugh score C	9 (45)	10 (50)		
Duration since diagnosis with advanced stage (days) [##]			1.245	0.776
≤30	4 (20)	6 (30)		
31–60	8 (40)	5 (25)		
61–90	5 (25)	5 (25)		
>90	3 (15)	4 (20)		

[#] Pearson Chi-square test [##] Fisher's exact test.

Table 3. Comparison of anxiety and depression scores at baseline between experimental and control groups (N = 40).

Variables	Group	Mean	SD	df	t	p-Value
Anxiety	Experiment	10.65	0.67	19	0.24	0.813
	Control	10.70	0.65			
Depression	Experiment	10.40	0.82	19	1.59	0.119
	Control	9.70	1.78			

Following the intervention program, the experimental group's mean scores for anxiety and depression decreased significantly at post-test compared to baseline (Table 4).

Table 4. Comparison of anxiety and depression scores at each point of measurement in experimental group (n = 20).

Variables	Time Point	Mean	SD	df	t	p-Value
Anxiety						
	Pretest	10.65	0.67	19	7.55	0.000 *
	Post-test	9.15	0.81			
Depression						
	Pretest	10.40	0.82	19	5.44	0.000 *
	Post-test	8.80	1.10			

* $p < 0.001$.

The post-test comparison between the experimental and control groups found that the mean scores for anxiety and depression in the experimental group were significantly lower than those of the control group (Table 5).

Table 5. Comparisons of anxiety and depression scores after intervention between experimental and control groups (N = 40).

Variables	Group	Mean	SD	df	t	p-Value
Anxiety	Experiment	9.15	0.81	38	4.05	0.000 *
	Control	10.15	0.74			
Depression	Experiment	8.80	1.10	38	2.59	0.013 **
	Control	9.80	1.32			

* $p < 0.0001$, ** $p < 0.005$.

4. Discussion

This study was undertaken to evaluate the effectiveness of a program given to patients with advanced cancer and family caregivers for reducing anxiety and depression in patients. Hospitalized patients are apt to have high psychosocial distress, and family members are in a good position to influence that distress. Especially in Thailand, there is a large presence of family members in the hospital. Findings from this study demonstrated that the family involvement program reduced anxiety and depression in patients with advanced HCC. The program consisted of four aspects of family involvement, including health information sharing, care provision, decision making on treatments, and providing psychological support.

In this program, nurses were encouraged to build rapport and establish trusting relationships with patients and family during the first day of hospital admission. This is aimed at affirming an important role of families [28]. The nursing activities included encouraging patients and their caregivers to be open and share concerns as well as impacts of the cancer experiences on all family members. In the information sharing session, the nurse provided education and support tailored to patients' needs and preferences for the level of required information. She also invited family caregivers to participate and provided the booklet for patients and other family members to learn. Family members could help patients manage physical symptoms and cope with psychological concerns.

In addition, the nurse supported family members to engage in conversations with the physician. A previous study reported that health information assists patients in coping with the immediate and long-term physical, emotional, and social impacts of cancer [47].

Advance care planning is a key component of palliative care for patients with HCC [29]. Our nurse-led program facilitated family caregivers to become involved in decision making through providing and sharing information with the patient, coordinating care with medical doctors for consultation, and setting family meetings among the patient, family members, and healthcare providers. Patients often viewed their family members as supporters to help cope with cancer and treatment options and identify preferences [21] and mentioned that it was important to discuss or share any decisions made with their caregivers [48]. Therefore, these nursing activities would alleviate patients' psychological distress.

Another aspect of our nurse-led program was to encourage family caregivers to be involved in care provision. Based on PPS assessment, most of our study participants were in the transition phase. For the most part, these patients were unable to perform activities of daily living. Encouraging family caregivers to be involved in daily patient care such as bathing, grooming, or eating can fulfill the physical needs of their loved ones. Furthermore, during care involvement, patients and family caregivers spend time together, which can enhance the intimate relationship and promote a sense of connectedness and alleviate feelings of loneliness [40].

Our findings confirmed the previous systematic review, which reported that psycho-oncological intervention can alleviate depressive symptoms and anxiety in patients with HCC [6] and patients with prostate cancer [22,23] and with breast cancer [24,25]. This nurse-led program is appropriate for an inpatient setting. In general, the length of stay of hospitalized patients with HCC in the selected hospital was five to six days. Therefore, our brief one-on-one family involvement program could be beneficial for both health care providers and patients as well as their family. It can be provided during hospital visiting times each day. It has been reported that a brief intervention, delivered by lay persons, can promote adjustment among newly diagnosed cancer patients at high risk of developing anxiety or depressive disorders [49]. Nurses take roles to facilitate interaction and communication among patients, family, and health care providers. Based on our observations during implementation of the program, we witnessed happy moments and saw the sparking eyes among patients. Instead of lying on their beds all day, these patients looked energized. Our study participants also reflected that they spent their time together meaningfully. When all aspects of the intervention are provided in a synchronized manner, they can alleviate psychological distress as experienced by these patients.

5. Limitation of the Study

There are some limitations in this study. The participants were family caregivers of male patients with advanced HCC in the university hospital, Southern, Thailand. Therefore, generalization to other settings and female patients is limited. This study was conducted during the COVID-19 pandemic, hence there was a limited number of eligible participants in the study. It would be valuable to repeat the study with a larger sample as well as with a female patient sample. Finally, the outcomes were assessed immediately after the program completion. Interventions cannot be assumed to have long-term effects. Moreover, only patient outcomes were measured. Further studies should be undertaken to examine the outcomes on family caregivers and measure the outcomes over a more extended period in both patients and family caregivers. Due to the complexity of care demands among other hospitalized patients, implementing the program in other inpatient settings may require adjusting the intervention to make it more practical in real-world settings.

6. Conclusions and Implications

Depression and anxiety are common among patients with HCC. The study addressed the significance of family involvement in alleviating anxiety and depression in hospitalized patients with advanced HCC. The results show that our nurse-led family involvement program had a short-term effect of reducing anxiety and depression symptoms immediately after intervention. This program was delivered successfully by registered nurses to patients with moderate levels of psychosocial distress. In the future, to implement the program in medical settings, nurses will require preparation for screening psychological distress and providing the intervention through orientation to the program activities.

Author Contributions: Conceptualization, S.K., S.T., K.N., and M.I.F.; methodology, S.T., K.N., and M.I.F.; validation, S.K. and K.N.; intervention, S.K.; formal analysis, S.T; writing—original draft preparation, S.T., and K.N.; writing—review and editing, K.N. and M.I.F.; funding acquisition, S.T.; project administration, S.T. All authors have read and agreed to the published version of the manuscript.

Funding: This research was funded by the Faculty of Medicine Research Funds (grant number: 62-00015).

Institutional Review Board Statement: The Institutional Review Board of the Faculty of Medicine, Prince of Songkla University approval was obtained before the study was initiated (EC 62-131-15-7).

Informed Consent Statement: Informed consent was obtained from all subjects involved in the study.

Conflicts of Interest: The authors declare no conflict of interest.

References

1. Laube, R.; Sabih, A.H.; Strasser, S.I.; Lim, L.; Cigolini, M.; Liu, K. Palliative care in hepatocellular carcinoma. *J. Gastroenterol. Hepatol.* **2021**, *36*, 618–628. [CrossRef] [PubMed]
2. Chen, J.J.; Huang, S.S.; Li, I.F.; Lin, K.P.; Tsay, S.L. Prognostic association of demographic and clinical factors with the change rates of symptoms and depression among patients with hepatocellular carcinoma. *Support Care Cancer* **2019**, *27*, 4665–4674. [CrossRef] [PubMed]
3. Kumar, M.; Panda, D. Role of supportive care for terminal stage hepatocellular carcinoma. *J. Clin. Exp. Hepatol.* **2014**, *4* (Suppl. S3), S130–S139. [CrossRef] [PubMed]
4. Ayman, A.; Azza, A.; Kamel, Y.; Rasul, K.; Jonas, F.; Mohammed, A.; Zeinab, M. The role of palliative care in the management of patients with advanced hepatocellular carcinoma: A single institution experience. *J. Patient Care* **2017**, *2*, 1000112. [CrossRef]
5. Niedzwiedz, C.L.; Knifton, L.; Robb, K.A.; Katikireddi, S.V.; Smith, D.J. Depression and anxiety among people living with and beyond cancer: A growing clinical and research priority. *BMC Cancer* **2019**, *19*, 943. [CrossRef] [PubMed]
6. Graf, J.; Stengel, A. Psychological burden and psycho-oncological interventions for patients with hepatobiliary cancers–a systematic review. *Front Psychol.* **2021**, *12*, 662777. [CrossRef] [PubMed]
7. Chang, C.H.; Chen, S.J.; Liu, C.Y. Risk of developing depressive disorders following hepatocellular carcinoma: A nationwide population-based study. *PLoS ONE* **2015**, *10*, e0135417. [CrossRef]
8. Riedl, D.; Schüßler, G. Factors associated with and risk factors for depression in cancer patients - a systematic literature review. *Transl Oncol.* **2022**, *16*, 101328. [CrossRef]
9. Hart, N.H.; Crawford-Williams, F.; Crichton, M.; Yee, J.; Smith, T.J.; Koczwara, B.; Fitch, M.I.; Crawford, G.B.; Mukhopadhyay, S.; Mahony, J.; et al. Unmet supportive care needs of people with advanced cancer and their caregivers: A systematic scoping review. *Crit. Rev. Oncol. Hematol.* **2022**, *176*, 103728. [CrossRef]
10. Wang, T.; Molassiotis, A.; Chung, B.P.M.; Tan, J.Y. Unmet care needs of advanced cancer patients and their informal caregivers: A systematic review. *BMC Palliat Care* **2018**, *17*, 96. [CrossRef]
11. National Cancer Institute. *Hospital-Based Cancer Registry*; 2021. Available online: https://www.nci.go.th/e_book/hosbased_2564/index.html (accessed on 5 December 2022).
12. Somboon, K.; Siramolpiwat, S.; Vilaichone, R.K. Epidemiology and survival of hepatocellular carcinoma in the central region of Thailand. *Asian Pac. J. Cancer Prev.* **2014**, *15*, 3567–3570. [CrossRef] [PubMed]
13. Temtap, S.; Nilmanat, K. The relationship between psychological distress and coping strategies in patients with advanced or terminal stage hepatocellular carcinoma: A cross-sectional descriptive study. *Songklanagarind Med. J.* **2017**, *35*, 313. [CrossRef]
14. Weis, J. Psychosocial Care for Cancer Patients. *Breast Care (Basel)* **2015**, *10*, 84–86. [CrossRef] [PubMed]
15. Wang, J.; Yan, C.; Fu, A. A randomized clinical trial of comprehensive education and care program compared to basic care for reducing anxiety and depression and improving quality of life and survival in patients with hepatocellular carcinoma who underwent surgery. *Medicine (Baltimore)* **2019**, *98*, e17552. [CrossRef]
16. Aprilianto, E.; Lumadi, S.A.; Handian, F.I. Family social support and the self-esteem of breast cancer patients undergoing neoadjuvant chemotherapy. *J. Public Health Res.* **2021**, *10*, jphr-2021. [CrossRef]

17. Moghaddam Tabrizi, F.; Alizadeh, S. Family intervention based on the FOCUS program effects on cancer coping in Iranian breast cancer patients: A Randomized Control Trial. *Asian Pac. J. Cancer. Prev.* **2018**, *19*, 1523–1528. [CrossRef]
18. Sari, D.K.; Dewi, R.; Daulay, W. Association between family support, coping strategies and anxiety in cancer patients undergoing chemotherapy at general hospital in Medan, North Sumatera, Indonesia. *Asian Pac. J. Cancer Prev.* **2019**, *20*, 3015–3019. [CrossRef]
19. Hopkinson, J.B.; Brown, J.C.; Okamoto, I.; Addington-Hall, J.M. The effectiveness of patient-family carer (couple) intervention for the management of symptoms and other health-related problems in people affected by cancer: A systematic literature search and narrative review. *J. Pain Symptom Manage* **2012**, *43*, 111–142. [CrossRef]
20. Gwaza, E.; Msiska, G. Family involvement in caring for inpatients in acute care hospital settings: A systematic review of literature. *SAGE Open Nurs.* **2022**, *8*, 23779608221089541. [CrossRef]
21. Dijkman, B.L.; Luttik, M.L.; Van der Wal-Huisman, H.; Paans, W.; van Leeuwen, B.L. Factors influencing family involvement in treatment decision-making for older patients with cancer: A scoping review. *J. Geriatr. Oncol.* **2022**, *13*, 391–397. [CrossRef]
22. Chien, C.H.; Liu, K.L.; Chien, H.T.; Liu, H.E. The effects of psychosocial strategies on anxiety and depression of patients diagnosed with prostate cancer: A systematic review. *Int. J. Nurs. Stud.* **2014**, *51*, 28–38. [CrossRef]
23. Newby, T.A.; Graff, J.N.; Ganzini, L.K.; McDonagh, M.S. Interventions that may reduce depressive symptoms among prostate cancer patients: A systematic review and meta-analysis. *Psychooncology* **2015**, *24*, 1686–1693. [CrossRef]
24. Guarino, A.; Polini, C.; Forte, G.; Favieri, F.; Boncompagni, I.; Casagrande, M. The effectiveness of psychological treatments in women with breast cancer: A systematic review and meta-analysis. *J. Clin. Med.* **2020**, *9*, 209. [CrossRef]
25. Xiao, F.; Song, X.; Chen, Q.; Dai, Y.; Xu, R.; Qiu, C.; Guo, Q. Effectiveness of psychological interventions on depression in patients after breast cancer surgery: A meta-analysis of randomized controlled trials. *Clin. Breast Cancer* **2017**, *17*, 171–179. [CrossRef] [PubMed]
26. Kamaryati, N.P.; Malathum, P. Family support: A concept analysis. *PRIJNR* **2020**, *24*, 403–411.
27. Coyne, E.; Heynsbergh, N.; Dieperink, K.B. Acknowledging cancer as a family disease: A systematic review of family care in the cancer setting. *Eur. J. Oncol. Nurs.* **2020**, *49*, 101841. [CrossRef] [PubMed]
28. Laidsaar-Powell, R.; Butow, P.; Boyle, F.; Juraskova, I. Facilitating collaborative and effective family involvement in the cancer setting: Guidelines for clinicians (TRIO Guidelines-1). *Patient Educ. Couns.* **2018**, *101*, 970–982. [CrossRef]
29. Virdun, C.; Luckett, T.; Davidson, P.M.; Phillips, J. Dying in the hospital setting: A systematic review of quantitative studies identifying the elements of end-of-life care that patients and their families rank as being most important. *Palliat. Med.* **2015**, *29*, 774–796. [CrossRef]
30. Hobbs, G.S.; Landrum, M.B.; Arora, N.K.; Ganz, P.A.; van Ryn, M.; Weeks, J.C.; Mack, J.W.; Keating, N.L. The role of families in decisions regarding cancer treatments. *Cancer* **2015**, *121*, 1079–1087. [CrossRef]
31. Hien, L.T.; Chanruangvanich, W.; Thosingha, O. Factors related to needs in palliative care among patients with hepatocellular carcinoma. *Nurs. Sci. J. Thail* **2017**, *35*, 87–95.
32. Woodrell, C.D.; Hansen, L.; Schiano, T.D.; Goldstein, N.E. Palliative care for people with hepatocellular carcinoma, and specific benefits for older adults. *Clin. Ther.* **2018**, *40*, 512–525. [CrossRef] [PubMed]
33. Harris, E.; Eng, D.; Ang, Q.; Clarke, E.; Sinha, A. Goals of care discussions in acute hospital admissions-qualitative description of perspectives from patients, family and their doctors. *Patient Educ. Couns.* **2021**, *104*, 2877–2887. [CrossRef] [PubMed]
34. Wolff, J.L.; Roter, D.L. Family presence in routine medical visits: A meta-analytical review. *Soc. Sci. Med* **2011**, *72*, 823–831. [CrossRef]
35. Kaiser, K.; Mallick, R.; Butt, Z.; Mulcahy, M.F.; Benson, A.B.; Cella, D. Important and relevant symptoms including pain concerns in hepatocellular carcinoma (HCC): A patient interview study. *Support Care Cancer* **2014**, *22*, 919–926. [CrossRef]
36. Li, L.; Mo, F.K.; Chan, S.L.; Hui, E.P.; Tang, N.S.; Koh, J.; Leung, L.K.S.; Poon, A.N.Y.; Hui, J.; Chu, C.M.; et al. Prognostic values of EORTC QLQ-C30 and QLQ-HCC18 index-scores in patients with hepatocellular carcinoma-clinical application of health-related quality-of-life data. *BMC Cancer* **2017**, *17*, 8. [CrossRef] [PubMed]
37. Ozdemir, S.; Malhotra, C.; Teo, I.; Tan, S.N.G.; Wong, W.H.M.; Joad, A.S.K.; Hapuara, T.; Gayatri, P.; Tuong, P.N.; Bhatnagar, S.; et al. Patient-reported roles in decision-making among Asian patients with advanced cancer: A multicountry study. *MDM Policy Pract.* **2021**, *6*, 23814683211061398. [CrossRef]
38. Christie, K.M.; Meyerowitz, B.E.; Giedzinska-Simons, A.; Gross, M.; Agus, D.B. Predictors of affect following treatment decision-making for prostate cancer: Conversations, cognitive processing, and coping. *Psychooncology* **2009**, *18*, 508–514. [CrossRef]
39. Kvåle, K. Do cancer patients always want to talk about difficult emotions? A qualitative study of cancer inpatients communication needs. *Eur. J. Oncol. Nurs.* **2007**, *11*, 320–327. [CrossRef]
40. Zeilani, R.S.; Abdalrahim, M.S.; Hamash, K.; Albusoul, R.M. The experience of family support among patients newly diagnosed with cancer in Jordan. *Eur. J. Oncol. Nurs.* **2022**, *60*, 102173. [CrossRef]
41. Des Jarlais, D.C.; Lyles, C.; Crepaz, N. Improving the reporting quality of nonrandomized evaluations of behavioral and public health interventions: The TREND statement. *Am. J. Public Health* **2004**, *94*, 361–366. [CrossRef]
42. Nilchaikovit, T.; Lortrakul, M.; Phisansuthideth, U. Development of Thai version of Hospital Anxiety and Depression Scale in cancer patients. *J. Psychiatr. Assoc. Thailand* **1996**, *41*, 18–30.
43. Polit, D.F.; Beck, C.T. *Nursing Research: Principles and Methods*, 7th ed.; Lippincott Williams and Wilkins: Philadelphia, PA, USA, 2003.

44. Chewaskulyong, B.; Sapinun, L.; Downing, G.M.; Intaratat, P.; Lesperance, M.; Leautrakul, S.; Somwangprasert, T.; Leerapun, T. Reliability and validity of the Thai translation (Thai PPS Adult Suandok) of the Palliative Performance Scale (PPSv2). *Palliat. Med.* **2012**, *26*, 1034–1041. [CrossRef] [PubMed]
45. Tsoris, A.; Marlar, C.A. Use of the Child Pugh score in liver disease. In *StatPearls*; StatPearls Publishing Copyright © 2023; StatPearls Publishing LLC.: Treasure Island, FL, USA, 2022.
46. Zigmond, A.S.; Snaith, R.P. The hospital anxiety and depression scale. *Acta Psychiatr. Scand* **1983**, *67*, 361–370. [CrossRef] [PubMed]
47. McCorkle, R.; Ercolano, E.; Lazenby, M.; Schulman-Green, D.; Schilling, L.S.; Lorig, K.; Wagner, E.H. Self-management: Enabling and empowering patients living with cancer as a chronic illness. *CA Cancer J. Clin.* **2011**, *61*, 50–62. [CrossRef] [PubMed]
48. Cincidda, C.; Pizzoli, S.F.M.; Ongaro, G.; Oliveri, S.; Pravettoni, G. Caregiving and shared decision making in breast and prostate cancer patients: A systematic review. *Curr. Oncol.* **2023**, *30*, 803–823. [CrossRef]
49. Pitceathly, C.; Maguire, P.; Fletcher, I.; Parle, M.; Tomenson, B.; Creed, F. Can a brief psychological intervention prevent anxiety or depressive disorders in cancer patients? A randomised controlled trial. *Ann. Oncol.* **2009**, *20*, 928–934. [CrossRef]

Disclaimer/Publisher's Note: The statements, opinions and data contained in all publications are solely those of the individual author(s) and contributor(s) and not of MDPI and/or the editor(s). MDPI and/or the editor(s) disclaim responsibility for any injury to people or property resulting from any ideas, methods, instructions or products referred to in the content.

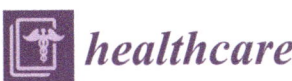

Article

Perspectives on Emotional Care: A Qualitative Study with Cancer Patients, Carers, and Health Professionals

Meinir Krishnasamy [1,2,3,4,*], Heidi Hassan [1], Carol Jewell [2], Irene Moravski [2,3] and Tennille Lewin [1,2,5]

1 Academic Nursing Unit, Peter MacCallum Cancer Centre, Melbourne, VIC 3000, Australia
2 Department of Nursing, School of Health Sciences, University of Melbourne, Melbourne, VIC 3052, Australia
3 Victorian Comprehensive Cancer Centre Alliance, Melbourne, VIC 3000, Australia
4 Sir Peter MacCallum Department of Oncology, University of Melbourne, Melbourne, VIC 3052, Australia
5 Department of Epidemiology and Preventive Medicine, Monash University, Melbourne, VIC 3168, Australia
* Correspondence: meinir.krishnasamy@petermac.org

Abstract: The emotional consequences of a cancer diagnosis are well documented and range from emotional distress, defined as suffering associated with feelings such as shock, fear, and uncertainty, through to psychological distress that may manifest as depression, anxiety, feelings of hopelessness, or heightened risk of suicide. This study set out to explore the assumption that the provision of emotional care should be the platform upon which all other aspects of cancer care are delivered and, that without attention to emotional care, no other aspects of cancer care can be fully realized. Utilizing qualitative focus groups and in-depth interviews with 47 patients, carers, and health professionals, emotional care was shown to be (1) fundamental to the provision of comprehensive cancer care, (2) essential to easing the burden of a cancer diagnosis and demands of treatment, (3) everyone's business, and (4) a component of cancer care at any time and every time. Future studies are needed to test interventions to enhance provision of intentional, purposeful, and individualized emotional care to help patents achieve the best health outcomes possible.

Keywords: cancer care; emotional care; person-centered care; qualitative research

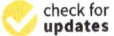

Citation: Krishnasamy, M.; Hassan, H.; Jewell, C.; Moravski, I.; Lewin, T. Perspectives on Emotional Care: A Qualitative Study with Cancer Patients, Carers, and Health Professionals. *Healthcare* 2023, 11, 452. https://doi.org/10.3390/healthcare11040452

Academic Editor: Reza Mortazavi

Received: 30 December 2022
Revised: 29 January 2023
Accepted: 2 February 2023
Published: 4 February 2023

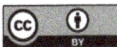

Copyright: © 2023 by the authors. Licensee MDPI, Basel, Switzerland. This article is an open access article distributed under the terms and conditions of the Creative Commons Attribution (CC BY) license (https://creativecommons.org/licenses/by/4.0/).

1. Introduction

Cancer and its treatments can affect every aspect of an individual's life, giving rise to a range of supportive care needs that can include informational, physical, practical, social, spiritual, psychological, and emotional requirements [1]. When left unaddressed, these needs can impact capacity to tolerate or adhere to treatment, capacity to engage in treatment decision-making, patient experience and health outcomes, and health system costs [2,3]. Supportive care refers to the provision of services, resources, and interventions required by people to cope with the needs triggered or exacerbated by a diagnosis of cancer, the demands of treatment, and ongoing consequences of a cancer diagnosis [1] and is recognized as a component of quality cancer care [4]. This paper reports on experiences of emotional care as a distinct component of supportive care, as reported by people affected by cancer and health care professionals involved in their care. The data were collected as part of a larger study (described below). The manuscript is not concerned with provision of psychological care for patients who present with or develop complex mental health issues during a cancer experience, which require specialist psychological or psychiatric intervention.

Cancer, Supportive Care, and Emotional Health

The emotional health consequences of a cancer diagnosis have been well documented and range from emotional distress (suffering associated with feelings such as shock, fear, and uncertainty), through to psychological distress that may manifest as depression, anxiety, feelings of hopelessness, or heightened risk of suicide [5,6]. Approximately 35–40% of patients with cancer experience emotional or psychological distress at some stage during their illness [7,8], and this is especially so for patients who enter the health system already burdened by poverty, poor health literacy, rurality, cultural and linguistic diversity, or who belong to Indigenous or First Nations peoples [9]. Emotional care refers to the identification of and tailored responses to the emotional suffering experienced by people affected by cancer [1].

Furthermore, people affected by some cancers, such as head and neck cancer, are estimated to have suicide rates up to four times higher compared with the general population [10]. Cancer caregivers also experience considerable unmet emotional need, especially when the trajectory of care is prolonged [11] or where prognosis is poor at time at diagnosis [12]. Indeed, several studies have demonstrated that caregivers experience more emotional challenges than patients themselves [13,14]. Combined, patients with advanced cancers and their carers report emotional and psychological needs as the most prevalent unmet supportive care domains [12].

Although timely, targeted, and personalized supportive care screening, assessment, and intervention has been shown to relieve emotional and psychological needs following a cancer diagnosis [15–17], provision of supportive care (and thus attention to emotional and psychological needs) remains inconsistent [18]. This is concerning given evidence demonstrates that the emotional wellbeing of patients is linked to their ability to communicate with members of their health care team, make decisions, adhere to treatment, and achieve optimal physical health outcomes [19]. One explanation for this may be the conceptualization of emotional care (as a component of supportive care) as something adjunct or additive to the treatment of cancer care [20], rather than recognizing it as the platform upon which all other aspects of cancer care should be constructed or delivered [4].

The data reported in this paper are drawn from a large mixed-methods study undertaken to refresh and develop new approaches to the integration of cancer supportive care as a component of routine cancer service delivery. The study was funded by the Victorian Department of Health in Australia and approved by the University of Melbourne Human Research Ethics Committee (ID REF: 185 1227.5). A broad community of 300 cancer consumers (patients/family members/support persons), health professionals, health services researchers, policy makers, and not for profit organization members (other participants) took part in the mixed methods study, and data gathered were used to build an online supportive care portal (https://wecan.org.au (accessed on 20 December 2022).) (publication in preparation). Here, we present insights gained from qualitative focus groups and in-depth interviews undertaken as part of the larger study between January–November 2018 regarding provision of emotional care. This paper sets out to report participants' accounts of experiencing or responding to emotional distress, as defined above. It also sets out to consider whether data generated support the assumption that the provision of emotional care should be the platform upon which all other aspects of cancer care are delivered and, that without attention to emotional care, no other aspects of cancer care can be fully realized.

2. Materials and Methods

An exploratory qualitative approach, utilizing data collected during Town Hall and Community of Practice events as part of the larger mixed methods study. Town Hall meetings are a recognized approach to community engagement when a broad and inclusive approach to data collection is required to meet study aims [21]. A Community of Practice is a group of people who come together over a period of time to share an interest in, address, and learn more about a particular topic [22].

2.1. Methods

Focus groups were chosen to collect data during the larger supportive care study, to facilitate interaction among a large and diverse group of participants, in order to generate a wide range of views and ideas [23]. Participants who were unable to attend a focus group were offered the opportunity to take part in an in-depth interview.

2.2. Recruitment and Consent

Recruitment involved purposive and snowball sampling techniques [24]. Initially, a list of key stakeholders (described above as part of the larger mixed methods study) was developed by the project lead who had experience of and expertise in cancer supportive care (MK). The aim was to purposively recruit a diverse sample of participants with experience of supportive care either as a cancer patient, carer (i.e., family member or informal support person), or health professional. Potential participants were approached directly via email describing the intent of the study and inviting them to take part. The email contained a flyer explaining eligibility criteria, what participation would involve, and details of how to contact a member of the project team to express interest in taking part. Potential participants were asked to forward on the flyer to colleagues/friends they believed met the eligibility criteria and who might be interested in taking part. Eligibility criteria for people affected by cancer were: (1) current or previous cancer diagnosis or family member/support person of somebody who has/had a cancer diagnosis, (2) 18 years of age or over, (3) able to provide informed consent, and (4) able to read, write and speak English or take part with support of a family member/support person. Eligibility criteria for the health professionals were: (1) experience of working with/supporting people affected by cancer in any aspect of the health sector, (2) 18 years of age or over, and (3) able to provide informed consent. Following contact with a member of the project team (MK, IM, CJ), a copy of the Participant Information and Consent Form (PICF) was emailed or mailed to participants to read and sign and bring it along with them on the day of the focus group or interview. Participants who took part in an interview remotely (that is via telephone) were asked to return the signed consent form via email or mail, as preferred. Consent was also re-checked verbally and audio-recorded on the day of the focus group or interview.

2.3. Data Collection

After re-checking consent at the beginning of each focus group or interview, participants were asked to complete a brief demographic data collection form to indicate their status as a patient, carer, or health professional, their age, place of residence or work, language spoken at home (patients and carers) or, their professional affiliation (health professionals only). Intentionally, no data on cancer diagnosis, time since treatment completion, or treatments received were collected from patients or carers as there was no intention to undertake any tests of association or to consider experiences of emotional care in the context of a specific diagnosis. As such, collecting these data seemed intrusive. To address any potential imbalance of power by having health professionals, patients, and carers in the same focus groups [25], three patient and carer, and three health professional focus groups were conducted separately. Of the six focus groups, two were held in a regional setting, ensuring that the study was accessible to people affected by cancer and health professionals outside of metropolitan sites. Patient and carer participants were compensated for their travel and parking cost. Focus groups were moderated by two members of the project team (MK, CJ, IM), one to lead discussion and a second to observe and take notes of context and environment and to ensure that all participants had an opportunity to contribute. Interviews were conducted by the same project team members. A semi-structured discussion guide (see Supplemental Material S1) was developed based on data generated by Town Hall meetings and Community of Practice events undertaken as part of the larger mixed methods study. The discussion guide facilitated exploration of participants' experiences and understanding of supportive care and their views of its value and importance. The questions did not specifically direct participants to emotional domains of supportive care and so the findings reported below represent spontaneous insights recounted by participants of their experiences and views regarding emotional care. An example of questions included in the focus groups and in-depth interviews is presented in Table 1. A full list of focus group and interview questions are available as Supplementary Material S1.

Table 1. Examples of focus group/interview questions.

Exploratory Questions
What does the term supportive care mean to you?
Can you think of a time you have had a positive "supportive care" experience?
What skills and experience do you think clinicians working with people affected by cancer need to have?
What do you think is most important or valuable about supportive care?

Interviews and focus groups were audio recorded and transcribed verbatim as word documents. Word documents were uploaded to NVivo 12 [26] to help organize and manage the analytical process. All study data were stored in secure electronic folders and only named members of the project team had access to audio-recordings, participants demographic data, and consent forms. Transcribed audio recordings were de-identified.

2.4. Analysis

Data analysis was undertaken in accordance with Braun and Clarke's six steps of thematic analysis [27]. Recordings from each data set were initially listened through, transcripts read, and notes made about general observations and impressions, as part of researcher familiarization and rich engagement with the data. Transcripts were coded by two independent coders (CJ, SM) and any disagreement clarified through discussion with the project lead (MK). A threshold for saturation was agreed prior to data analysis which was agreed as the point at which no new themes were generated through the analytical process. The focus was on producing semantic, rather than latent themes as a means of establishing a detailed description of the data, but without engaging in broader interpretative theorizing [28]. All data were coded line by line using an inductive process. Candidate themes were identified by reviewing the codes and individual codes were collated under candidate themes. Themes were refined and revised using a reflexive process, and consistent with Braun and Clarke's model, themes were conceptualized as constructs rather than representative of "reality" [28]. Participants' demographic data were analyzed descriptively. The manuscript has been prepared according to the Consolidated Criteria for Reporting Qualitative Research Checklist [29].

3. Results

3.1. Participants

Forty-seven participants (16 patients, six carers, and 25 health professionals) took part across six focus groups and eight interviews (Table 2).

Table 2. Participant demographics (n = 47).

Characteristics	Patients and Carers (n = 22)
Female	21 (95%)
Age (median and range)	63 (44–86)
Patient	16 (72%)
Family member/carer	6 (28%)
Place of residence	
Metropolitan	14 (64%)
Regional	7 (32%)
Not specified	1 (5%)
Language spoken at home	
English	100%

Table 2. *Cont.*

Characteristics	Health care participants (n = 25)
Male	3 (11%)
Female	22 (89%)
Age (median and range)	49 (27–63)
Profession	
Nurse	10 (36%)
Dietician	4 (14%)
Medical oncologist	3 (10%)
Psychologist	2 (7%)
Social Worker	1 (4%)
Physiotherapist	1 (4%)
Exercise physiologist	1 (4%)
Counsellor	1 (4%)
Radiation Therapist	1 (4%)
Clinical Trials Coordinator	1 (4%)
Place of work	
Metropolitan	15 (60%)
Regional	8 (29%)
Rural	2 (7%)

3.2. Focus Groups/Interviews

Four themes were generated that related to emotional care. No themes were unique to either focus group or interview participants. Themes are illustrated below by inclusion of participant quotes. Where more than one quote is included per theme, is it to illustrate nuance within the theme, rather than being indicative of a theme's prevalence within the data.

3.3. Emotional Care—A Fundamental Component of Cancer Care

People affected by cancer spoke of the provision of emotional care as being necessary to enable a person to live well, to cope throughout the treatment period, and beyond.

"So there's emotional care, there's physical care, there's managing symptoms of cancer and of treatment. The emotional support of the patient [is important] . . . so they can live well throughout that time." (P042)

Attending to a person's emotional needs was recognized by health professionals as fundamental to quality of life and ability to cope with the treatment "journey" and making it the best it could be.

"what . . . might be of benefit to that person, wherever they are in their treatment phase . . . what services . . . might be of benefit for them to improve quality of life, make their treatment better, make their journey better." (W FG HP01)

People affected by cancer spoke about their experience of emotional care in the context of help, advice, communication, and perhaps most significantly, listening and being responsive. Participants' emotional wellbeing was described as coming from feeling cared about, having a connection with a health professional who understood their struggles and circumstances, and took time to listen to them.

"The most important and valuable thing is I guess, yeah, it's that you've got someone to talk to about your emotional state. It's really about the emotional state I guess. It's having someone you can talk to about it, . . . your emotional feelings, just dealing with your anxieties and your emotions really." (PC046)

For some, this was a connection with a particular health professional, often a cancer nurse, while for others, this came through connections made in peer support groups and community services.

"it can be the simple things like, can I do the shopping or can I come and wash your dishes, and people don't know what to ask or how to ask if they could help." (M FG HP05)

For many health professionals ensuring access to practical support, delivered by nurses, occupational therapists, dietician, physiotherapists, psychologists, or social workers was regarded as an important emotional intervention where recognizing what a person needed practically, was a way of acknowledging an individual's unique circumstances, and a way of *'being with'* a person.

"For me it means it's other people to help so that the patient's got lots of experts to help them with all of the needs that they've got." (M FG HP01)

3.4. Easing the Burden

For many participants, the provision of emotional care was synonymous with easing the burden of a cancer diagnosis. Easing the burden came in very many forms, from ensuring that personal needs were attended to whilst in hospital, recognizing that someone is experiencing hardship and making it possible to ask for help, finding practical solutions to problems such as living arrangements, getting the shopping, knowing how to tell family about the diagnosis, and recognizing the mounting costs and financial concerns. These were all recognized as the provision of emotional care because they took account of the wider context of the person's life and the extensive impacts of a cancer diagnosis.

"[health professionals] need to not just look at us as a physical thing, they need to look at us as the whole person, they need to look at us how we are emotionally and especially in our situations outside, our family situations and work with that as well because that's what makes us get better and it's what makes us feel supported if they, you know, that they're involved and understand what's going on ... " (M FG CC 07)

People affected by cancer described being unclear about what support or help was on offer to them, especially soon after diagnosis, and there was a concern that people might miss out on important care as a consequence.

"if you say to a person do you want [support] or supportive care and they say no, what do they understand that they were gonna get, or what have they just missed out on." (PC041)

Health professionals spoke about the importance of being explicit about what was on offer, of asking gently probing questions to ensure that patients' needs were identified, and that they were made aware of what help was available to them. Taking a sensitive approach to asking the questions was recognized as an important component of emotional care, preventing people from feeling that they were "not coping" if they were having difficulties, especially when this related to issues of emotional need.

"I would just talk about whatever [service] it was. Like say, you know, it might be valuable to do this ... or it might be valuable for you to do this." (W FG HP03)

"I think that when you're trying to integrate a service that's got stigma attached to it or that people might feel ... , don't want to admit that, you know, they need extra help." (PC041)

Critical to easing the burden and the provision of emotional care was acknowledging people as individuals with unique and dynamic needs.

"it needs to be individualised. If you've got a child with cancer your needs are far different to what having a husband with cancer is, having cancer yourself, it's just got to be ... individualised, tailored." (R FG CC 011)

"I did ask, I'm really struggling, and maybe the staff could see that. So, you know, having staff at the hospitals that see that ... is pretty important." (PC046)

3.5. Emotional Care—Everyone's Business

The provision of emotional care was universally considered to be the responsibility of all health professionals. Having a person's concerns or needs respected or acknowledged, even if a clinician could not directly deal with them, was recognized as important to addressing a person's emotional wellbeing.

> "I think that concept of, you know, the word respect and taking the time to get to understand the person you're speaking with." (M FG HPC07)

> "You want them to have the attitude of this is about you, so we're gonna answer your questions and if I haven't got time to answer them now we're gonna organise a time where we're gonna sit down and we're gonna go through all your questions." (M FG PC08)

Communication skills were identified by almost every patient and carer as being essential to the provision of emotional care. Strategies such as making eye-contact, introducing oneself at the beginning of the consultation, using the patient's name, having read case notes prior to the consultation, and having an un-rushed manner were described as making the difference between feeling emotionally supported and recognized as a person, not just a patient.

> "People who come in ... and then they sit there with your notes and proceed to, um, ask you questions, and I have on one occasion had to tell a registrar you should be reading those notes prior to coming in to our consultation otherwise, um, our consultation is not going to be very meaningful .... So that sort of person I wouldn't talk to about my fear of recurrence for example because I would think they haven't even bothered to read the notes before walking in so what's their care factor." (PC049)

Many health professionals spoke of the need to introduce conversations that were about addressing emotional care with a lead-in, prefacing offers of support with an outline of the general concept of care that extends beyond medical treatment.

> "you have to preface it by saying I'm giving you this form to have a look at and complete because we know that we can provide you with extra services but we don't know specifically what we think you need." (PC040)

Some spoke of time taken to sit with someone in their distress, listen carefully to understand their needs, and ask gently probing questions as being an investment in avoiding difficulties escalating, or even reaching a crisis point before being addressed.

> "I think the biggest thing ... is ... it's actually having a conversation with the person ... actually sit down and ... you might refer them [there]." (M FG HP 010)

People affected by cancer and health professionals identified these components of care as being central to provision of emotional support. The ability to ask any health professional about their needs or concerns, and health professionals' willingness and ability help patients find the most appropriate support either directly or via a referral, were highly valued aspects of emotional care.

> "it's part of routine supportive care to actually do this identification of need ... to do that in a way that's palatable to patients, and in a way that facilitates ... them getting access to the right supports at the right time." (PC041)

However, complex barriers, such as lack of time to address emotional needs or having the skills required to initiate and manage emotional discussion, were acknowledged by all participants.

> "There's just that everyone is so very busy, so taking time to stop and actually think about what the patient might want or need is hard work ... especially ward nurses ... they're under such pressure. And then I think there's people that don't have the skills to ask those questions ... you know, some people are frightened to ask patients about how they're feeling properly because they are frightened they won't be able to deal with that or, you know, be able to help them once they tell them." (PC042)

The tension between demands on health professionals' time to meet large patient caseloads whilst having only a short amount of time allocated to each patient, was recognized.

"you don't want to be a burden ... you know people are busy" (MFG CC 03)

"so they [health professionals] would say yeah we're aware that patients are distressed, we're aware that it's a terrible time, but you know, we're trying to deal with their physical needs, we're trying to get through the tasks that are required to get them physically well." (P040)

3.6. Emotional Care—Anytime, Every Time

The provision of emotional care was recognized as fundamental to wellbeing across all stages of a person's cancer experience.

"I think the early stages is where a lot more supportive services should be in whether you want them or not, because the first thing's shock, grief, you know, who do I talk to, do I tell the kids, no I don't, do I or don't I and how do you tell them ... I think the end of life there's a lot more research done into dying and death and there's all that. It's that first three months is the hardest." (R FG CP 07)

For some participants the early stages of coming to terms with a diagnosis and engaging with treatment were felt to be so overwhelming that it was difficult to take anything else in and the importance of revisiting needs over time was highly valued.

"And even during treatment, so I had surgery and then chemotherapy and then radiotherapy, during most of that time I didn't really actively seek anything because I was so involved in just trying to get through my treatment." (PC046)

"this notion that ... just identify and then refer, it's short-sighted because things change and new things come up" (CP041)

The importance of continually screening for, assessing, and intervening (as appropriate) for emotional needs was emphasized by all patients and carers, emphasizing the dynamic nature of the emotional impost of a cancer diagnosis from diagnosis through to end of treatment and on into follow up care.

"once you've finished your active treatment, going back into the real world, you know, forming your new normal life, what's normal, because life has changed, and everyone looks at you like oh you're looking a lot better, your hair's grown back and you're looking healthy, so people think everything's fine but it's not because things have changed and you've got those fears and that sadness still there. So that's the crucial time where support's needed." (PC046)

However, irrespective of when support was provided, people affected by cancer were unanimous in their view that dedicated time and space was essential to enable meaningful emotional care, and that attention to emotional needs should be recognized as an intentional, purposeful, and distinct component of cancer care.

"I think it's difficult emotionally for patients to hold both sort of stances at once sometimes, to be thinking about the impact of their treatment on their life and what it means to them as a person, at the same time as trying to focus on the side effects of treatment and are those needs being addressed. I think having it separate, there is a role for that, even though we want of course all clinicians to have a certain level of understanding of [emotional care] and represent that in their practices." (CP041)

4. Discussion

This qualitative study explored insights from 47 people affected by cancer and health professionals through a series of six focus groups and eight in-depth interviews, that focused on perspectives of emotional care as a component of cancer care. Four key themes were generated focusing on, the centrality of emotional care within the concept of cancer care; the importance of easing the burden through intentional emotional care; emotional care as everyone's business; and the provision of emotional care as an enabler of emotional wellbeing across the entirety of a person's cancer experience.

The purpose of this paper was to explore the assumption that the provision of emotional care should be the platform upon which all other aspects of cancer care are delivered (emotional care anytime, every-time) and that without attention to emotional care, no other aspects of cancer care can be fully realized [4]. The paper set out to consider this assumption through perspectives of emotional care as recounted by patients with cancer, carers, and health professionals who had taken part in focus groups and in-depth interviews as part of a larger cancer supportive care study. Findings presented appear to support the assumption, whilst acknowledging that this is an initial exploratory study, representing insights from a predominantly female sample (patients and nurses) from metropolitan settings. As such, further research is needed to test this assumption more fully.

The importance of attending to the emotional stressors or burdens experienced following a cancer diagnosis has long been acknowledged, recognizing that cancer results in atypical levels of fear, worry, distress, and uncertainty for people affected by cancer [30]. Nevertheless, evidence demonstrates that the emotional needs of cancer patients (and those close to them) continue to be overlooked with damaging consequences such as inability to adhere to treatment [3,31,32]. This is not to suggest that cancer health care professionals lack care or empathy, but rather that they face considerable barriers within busy and often under-resourced health care settings to attend to needs beyond the cancer itself or to manage side-effects and symptoms of the treatment or the disease [30,33]. When integrated as the basis upon which cancer care is provided, actively asking about and listening to the needs of patients; empathy for their concerns; going beyond the minimum care provision required; timely identification and response to needs or concerns and, recognizing the needs of family members or carers have been described as powerful and practical ways to mitigate the emotional impost of cancer [30].

Our findings support many of these important insights. Our data demonstrate the importance placed by people affected by cancer and health professionals on the provision of emotional care and the creation of a safe emotional space where concerns and needs can be shared without fear of feeling a burden or as someone unable to cope. Skilled, empathic communication and the delivery of respectful person-centered care were identified as important components and enablers of emotional care and easing the burden. These are not new insights and are recognized as central tenets of patient centered care, benefits of which include enhanced patient experience, improved health outcomes, adherence to treatment, and improved health care costs [34], all of which have been shown to be sensitive outcomes to the provision of emotional care [15,16]. Consistent with other literature, our study demonstrated that the provision of emotional care is central to patients' experiences and outcomes of their cancer [35]. Our data also captured the importance of ensuring the availability of emotional care across the entirety of a person's cancer experience. Feeling able to talk to health professionals about emotional concerns, receiving information about services available, having needs acknowledged and validated by health professionals with the skills and knowledge to respond in a humane and respectful way, were critical to seeking and receiving impactful emotional care. These are important insights. With growing numbers of people being diagnosed with and living beyond cancer and its treatments [36,37], there is urgent need to enhance peoples' capacity to self-care (as they are able) to sustain their wellbeing through provision of timely emotional care. With a global health workforce shortage and reduction in health budgets in real terms [38–40], health systems will be unable to sustain the level of care currently provided to people with cancer. Enabling those who can access and proactively use emotional support services to do so will reduce burden on the health system, targeting scarce resources to those with greatest need for specialist emotional support and care. As health professionals there is opportunity for us to look outside acute health services and partner with not for profit, support, and advocacy groups who can deliver front line emotional care to people affected by cancer. Patients and carers in our study did not expect health professionals to have all the answers or resources to hand, indeed they were quick to recognize the limitations and burden on their time and capacity to deliver emotional care, but they did expect that health professionals would access or refer them to services available to meet their needs.

Patient and carer participants in this study noted that the absence of accessible emotional care resulted in feelings of isolation, of fear of missing out on care, and of being a patient in a system, rather than a person enveloped by support. Lack of information about where and how to access emotional support was described as exacerbating already complex situations, compounding feelings of isolation and fear, and provision of support without taking the time to understand a person's unique and dynamic needs potentially negated the opportunity for receipt of meaningful emotional care—impacting not only emotional wellbeing but cancer outcomes. Recently published evidence has demonstrated considerable return on investment for patients and health systems when patients receiving timely supportive care, inclusive of emotional care [2]. Our data support these findings, demonstrating advocacy for timely and ongoing access to emotional care for patients and carers, and investment in health professional knowledge and capability to deliver emotional care to prevent and mitigate the emotional impacts of a cancer diagnosis. Importantly, our data demonstrate that emotional care is a critical domain in the provision of cancer supportive care, requiring effective communication skill and empathy on the part of health professionals, and investment in time and resources by health services to enable and health professionals to deliver the care they recognize and value as components of patient-centered care.

An important insight from our study is that the provision of emotional care requires distinct and purposeful attention recognizing that it has to compete with the urgency of treating the cancer itself, " . . . *it's difficult emotionally for patients to hold both sort of stances at once sometimes, to be thinking about the impact of their treatment on their life and what it means to them as a person*". Participants in this study demonstrated the importance of creating an emotionally supportive context for the provision of the totality of cancer care, enabled through respectful interaction, provision of time and attention to individual needs, skilled communication and readiness to source and refer patients and carers to a diverse range of support services and resources.

The strengths of this study are that it generated data from a cohort of patients, carers, and health professionals with lived experience of providing and receiving cancer supportive care. The intent was not to generate generalizable data but to explore in-depth perspectives on emotional care as a component of cancer care. Data included participants living and working across metropolitan and regional areas of one state in Victoria, Australia. The paper provides novel insight on emotional care, offering insights to ways in which the experience of emotional care can be enhanced for consumers and enabled by health professionals. Future studies may focus on the impact of interventions to strengthen provision of emotional care, patient reports of care experiences, health outcomes, and system impacts. Insights from the focus groups and interviews were fed back to participants as part of the larger study. A key limitation of the study is that no people from Aboriginal or Torres Strait Islander or culturally or linguistically diverse peoples were included. As such, these findings are likely to present "the best' of experiences, and recommendations generated may have limited relevance to under-served populations.

5. Conclusions

In conclusion, emotional care is critical to the provision of patient-centered care, without which effective delivery of other aspects of cancer care may be hindered. The provision of emotional care and perceptions of its adequacy or impact rely on health professionals' communication skills; their ability to offer proactive opportunity for discussion of needs and concerns across all stages of the cancer experience, and importantly, their access to time and resources necessary to elicit and respond to emotional needs. For patients, availability of opportunity, encouragement to voice, and awareness of the legitimacy of emotional concerns are important facilitators of emotional care. Future studies are needed to test interventions to enhance provision of intentional and purposeful emotional care delivery to ensure patients achieve the best health outcomes possible. Studies focusing on the emotional care needs of underserved populations are urgently needed.

Supplementary Materials: The following supporting information can be downloaded at: https://www.mdpi.com/article/10.3390/healthcare11040452/s1, File S1: People affected by cancer: Focus group/interview schedule.

Author Contributions: Data curation, C.J.; Formal analysis, M.K., C.J.; Funding acquisition, M.K.; Investigation, C.J., I.M. and T.L.; Methodology, M.K. and T.L.; Project administration, M.K.; Supervision, M.K.; Writing—original draft, M.K. and H.H.; Writing—review and editing, C.J., I.M. and T.L. All authors have read and agreed to the published version of the manuscript.

Funding: This study was funded by the Victorian Department of Health, Australia.

Institutional Review Board Statement: The study was conducted in accordance with the Declaration of Helsinki, and approved by the University of Melbourne Human Research Ethics Committee ID REF: 185 1227.5 on 21 March 2018.

Informed Consent Statement: Informed consent was obtained from all subjects involved in the study.

Data Availability Statement: The data are stored electronically and in accordance with Good Clinical Practice requirements in the Academic Nursing Unit, The Peter MacCallum Cancer Centre, Melbourne Australia, De-identified data can be accessed from the lead author (MK).

Acknowledgments: The authors wish to acknowledge and sincerely thank all the participants who gave their time and expertise so generously to be part of this study. Thanks to Stella Mulder for her expert contribution to co-coding the data set from the larger study from which these data were extracted.

Conflicts of Interest: The authors confirm they have no individual, company or organization-based interests which involve financial or personal gain.

References

1. Fitch, M. Supportive care framework. *Can. Oncol. Nurs. J.* **2008**, *18*, 6–24. [CrossRef] [PubMed]
2. Hyatt, A.; Chung, H.; Aston, R.; Gough, K.; Krishnasamy, M. Social return on investment economic evaluation of supportive care for lung cancer patients in acute care settings in Australia. *BMC Health Serv. Res.* **2022**, *22*, 1399–1411. [CrossRef] [PubMed]
3. Zhu, L.; Tong, Y.X.; Xu, X.S.; Xiao, A.T.; Zhang, Y.J.; Zhang, S. High level of unmet needs and anxiety are associated with delayed initiation of adjuvant chemotherapy for colorectal cancer patients. *Support. Care Cancer* **2020**, *28*, 5299–5306. [CrossRef] [PubMed]
4. Krishnasamy, M.; Hyatt, A.; Chung, H.; Gough, K.; Fitch, M. Refocusing cancer supportive care: A framework for integrated cancer care. *Support. Care Cancer* **2022**, *31*, 14–24. [CrossRef] [PubMed]
5. Giedre, B.; Kamile, P. Interventions for reducing suicide risk in cancer patients: A literature review. *Eur. J. Psychol.* **2019**, *15*, 637–649.
6. Ferrari, M.; Ripamonti, C.I.; Hulbert-Williams, N.J.; Miccinesi, G. Relationships among unmet needs, depression, and anxiety in non-advanced cancer patients. *Tumori* **2019**, *105*, 144–150. [CrossRef]
7. Red Oak Recovery. Available online: https://www.redoakrecovery.com/addiction-blog/emotional-health-vs-mental-health (accessed on 28 December 2022).
8. McCarter, K.; Britton, B.; Baker, A.; Halpin, S.; Beck, A.; Carter, G.; Wratten, C.; Bauer, J.; Booth, D.; Forbes, E.; et al. Interventions to improve screening and appropriate referral of patients with cancer for distress: Systematic review protocol. *BMJ Open.* **2015**, *21*, e008277. [CrossRef]
9. Valery, P.C.; Bernardes, C.M.; Beesley, V.; Hawkes, A.L.; Baade, P.; Garvey, G. Unmet supportive care needs of Australian Aboriginal and Torres Strait Islanders with cancer: A prospective, longitudinal study. *Support. Care Cancer* **2017**, *25*, 869–877. [CrossRef]
10. Turner, K.; Stover, A.M.; Tometich, D.B.; Geiss, C.; Mason, A.; Nguyen, O.T.; Hume, E.; McCormick, R.; Powell, S.; Hallanger-Johnson, J.; et al. Oncology Providers' and Professionals' Experiences with Suicide Risk Screening among Patients with Head and Neck Cancer: A Qualitative Study. *JCO Oncol. Pract.* **2022**, OP2200433. [CrossRef]
11. Yang, W.F.Z.; Lee, R.Z.Y.; Kuparasundram, S.; Tan, T.; Chan, Y.H.; Griva, K.; Mahendran, R. Cancer caregivers unmet needs and emotional states across cancer treatment phases. *PLoS ONE* **2021**, *16*, e0255901. [CrossRef]
12. Hart, N.H.; Crawford-Williams, F.; Crichton, M.; Yee, J.; Smith, T.J.; Koczwara, B.; Fitch, M.I.; Crawford, G.B.; Mukhopadhyay, S.; Mahony, J.; et al. Unmet supportive care needs of people with advanced cancer and their caregivers: A systematic scoping review. *Crit. Rev. Oncol. Hematol.* **2022**, *176*, 103728. [CrossRef]
13. Kassir, Z.M.; Li, J.; Harrison, C.; Johnson, J.T.; Nilsen, M.L. Disparity of perception of quality of life between head and neck cancer patients and caregivers. *BMC Cancer* **2021**, *21*, 1127–1136. [CrossRef]

14. Haun, M.W.; Sklenarova, H.; Brechtel, A.; Herzog, W.; Hartmann, M. Distress in cancer patients and their caregivers and association with the caregivers' perception of dyadic communication. *Oncol. Res. Treat.* **2014**, *37*, 384–388. [CrossRef]
15. Hsieh, C.C.; Hsiao, F.H. The effects of supportive care interventions on depressive symptoms among patients with lung cancer: A metaanalysis of randomized controlled studies. *Palliat. Support. Care* **2017**, *15*, 710–723. [CrossRef]
16. Suh, S.R.; Lee, M.K. Effects of Nurse-Led Telephone-Based Supportive Interventions for Patients With Cancer: A Meta-Analysis. *Oncol. Nurs. Forum* **2017**, *44*, E168–E184. [CrossRef]
17. Erdoğan, Y.G.; Döner, A.; Muz, G. Psychological Distress and Its Association with Unmet Needs and Symptom Burden in Outpatient Cancer Patients: A Cross-Sectional Study. *Semin. Oncol. Nurs.* **2021**, *37*, 151–214. [CrossRef]
18. White, V.M.; Pejoski, N.; Vella, E.; Skaczkowski, G.; Ugalde, A.; Yuen, E.Y.N.; Livingston, P.; Wilson, C. Improving access to cancer information and supportive care services: A systematic review of mechanisms applied to link people with cancer to psychosocial supportive care services. *Psycho-Oncology* **2021**, *30*, 1603–1625. [CrossRef]
19. Gilmore, N.; Kehoe, L.; Bauer, J.; Xu, H.; Hall, B.; Wells, M.; Lei, L.; Culakova, E.; Flannery, M.; Grossman, V.A.; et al. The Relationship Between Frailty and Emotional Health in Older Patients with Advanced Cancer. *Oncologist* **2021**, *26*, e2181–e2191. [CrossRef]
20. Lubberding, S.; van Uden-Kraan, C.F.; Te Velde, E.A.; Cuijpers, P.; Leemans, C.R.; Verdonck-de Leeuw, I.M. Improving access to supportive cancer care through an eHealth application: A qualitative needs assessment among cancer survivors. *J. Clin. Nurs.* **2015**, *24*, 1367–1379. [CrossRef]
21. Etchegary, H.; Bishop, L.; Street, C.; Aubrey-Bassler, K.; Humphries, D.; Vat, L.E.; Barrett, B. Engaging patients in health research: Identifying research priorities through community town halls. *BMC Health Serv. Res.* **2017**, *17*, 192–199. [CrossRef]
22. Wenger, E.; Blackmore, C. Communities of practice and social learning systems: The career of a concept. In *Social Learning Systems and Communities of Practice*; Springer: London, UK, 2010; pp. 179–199.
23. Krueger, R.A.; Casey, M.A. *Focus Groups: A Practical Guide for Applied Research*; Sage Publication: Thousand Oaks, CA, USA, 2015.
24. Kandola, D.; Banner, D.; O'Keefe-McCarthy, S.; Jassal, D. Sampling Methods in Cardiovascular Nursing Research: An Overview. *Can. J. Cardiovasc. Nurs.* **2014**, *24*, 15–18. [PubMed]
25. The King's Fund Experience-Based Co-Design Toolkit. Available online: https://www.kingsfund.org.uk/projects/ebcd (accessed on 20 December 2022).
26. QSR International Pty Ltd. NVivo (Version 12, 2018). Available online: https://www.qsrinternational.com/nvivo-qualitative-data-analysis-software/home (accessed on 20 December 2022).
27. Braun, V.; Clarke, V. Using thematic analysis in psychology. *Quale. Res. Psych.* **2006**, *3*, 77–101. [CrossRef]
28. Braun, V.; Clarke, V. *Successful Qualitative Research: A Practical Guide for Beginner*; Sage Publication: Thousand Oaks, CA, USA, 2013.
29. Tong, A.; Sainsbury, P.; Craig, J. Consolidated criteria for reporting qualitative research (COREQ): A 32-item checklist for interviews and focus groups. *Int. J. Qual. Health Care* **2007**, *6*, 349–357. [CrossRef] [PubMed]
30. Kelley, J.M.; Kraft-Todd, G.; Schapira, L.; Kossowsky, J.; Riess, H. The influence of the patient-clinician relationship on healthcare outcomes: A systematic review and meta-analysis of randomized controlled trials. *PLoS ONE* **2014**, *9*, e94207. [CrossRef] [PubMed]
31. Schmidt, M.E.; Goldschmidt, S.; Hermann, S.; Steindorf, K. Late effects, long-term problems and unmet needs of cancer survivors. *Int. J. Cancer* **2022**, *151*, 1280–1290. [CrossRef]
32. Wang, T.; Molassiotis, A.; Chung, B.P.M.; Tan, J.Y. Unmet care needs of advanced cancer patients and their informal caregivers: A systematic review. *BMC Palliat. Care* **2018**, *17*, 96. [CrossRef]
33. Berry, L.L.; Danaher, T.S.; Chapman, R.A.; Awdish, R.L.A. Role of Kindness in Cancer Care. *J. Oncol. Pract.* **2017**, *13*, 744–750. [CrossRef]
34. Santana, M.; Ahmed, S.; Lorenzetti, D.; Jolley, R.J.; Manalili, K.; Zelinsky, S.; Quan, H.; Lu, M. Measuring patient-centred system performance: A scoping review of patient-centred care quality indicators. *BMJ Open.* **2019**, *9*, e023596. [CrossRef]
35. Prip, A.; Møller, K.A.; Nielsen, D.L.; Jarden, M.; Olsen, M.H.; Danielsen, A.K. The Patient-Healthcare Professional Relationship and Communication in the Oncology Outpatient Setting: A Systematic Review. *Cancer Nurs.* **2018**, *4*, E11–E22. [CrossRef]
36. Sung, H.; Ferlay, J.; Siegel, R.L.; Laversanne, M.; Soerjomataram, I.; Jemal, A.; Bray, F. Global Cancer Statistics 2020: GLOBOCAN Estimates of Incidence and Mortality Worldwide for 36 Cancers in 185 Countries. *CA Cancer J. Clin.* **2021**, *71*, 209–249. [CrossRef]
37. Lisy, K.; Langdon, L.; Piper, A.; Jefford, M. Identifying the most prevalent unmet needs of cancer survivors in Australia: A systematic review. *Asia-Pac. J. Clin. Oncol.* **2019**, *15*, e68–e78. [CrossRef]
38. Challinor, J.M.; Alqudimat, M.R.; Teixeira, T.O.A.; Oldenmenger, W.H. Oncology nursing workforce: Challenges, solutions, and future strategies. *Lancet Oncol.* **2020**, *21*, e564–e574. [CrossRef]
39. Mathew, A. Global Survey of Clinical Oncology Workforce. *J. Glob. Oncol.* **2018**, *4*, 1–12. [CrossRef]
40. Maruthappu, M.; Watkins, J.A.; Waqar, M.; Williams, C.; Ali, R.; Atun, R.; Faiz, O.; Zeltner, T. Unemployment, public-sector health-care spending and breast cancer mortality in the European Union: 1990–2009. *Eur. J. Public Health* **2015**, *25*, 330–335. [CrossRef]

Disclaimer/Publisher's Note: The statements, opinions and data contained in all publications are solely those of the individual author(s) and contributor(s) and not of MDPI and/or the editor(s). MDPI and/or the editor(s) disclaim responsibility for any injury to people or property resulting from any ideas, methods, instructions or products referred to in the content.

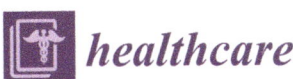

Article

Development of a Scale of Nurses' Competency in Anticipatory Grief Counseling for Caregivers of Patients with Terminal Cancer

Chia-Chi Hsiao [1,2,3], Suh-Ing Hsieh [4,5,*], Chen-Yi Kao [6] and Tsui-Ping Chu [1,3]

1. Department of Nursing, Chiayi Chang Gung Memorial Hospital, Chiayi County 61363, Taiwan
2. College of Nursing, Taipei Medical University, Taipei City 11031, Taiwan
3. Department of Nursing, Chang Gung University of Science and Technology Chiayi Campus, Chiayi County 61363, Taiwan
4. Department of Nursing, Chang Gung University of Science and Technology, Taoyuan City 33303, Taiwan
5. Department of Nursing, Taoyuan Chang Gung Memorial Hospital, Taoyuan City 33378, Taiwan
6. Hospice and Palliative Care Ward, Taoyuan Chang Gung Memorial Hospital, Taoyuan City 33353, Taiwan
* Correspondence: ishsieh@mail.cgust.edu.tw; Tel.: +886-3-2118999 (ext. 3423)

Abstract: Anticipatory grief leads to a highly stressful and conflicting experience among caregivers of patients with terminal cancer. Nurses lack the competency to assess and manage the caregivers' psychological problems, which in turn affects the caregivers' quality of life. A scale assessing the anticipatory grief counseling competency among nurses is unavailable. In this study, an Anticipatory Grief Counseling Competency Scale (AGCCS) was developed for nurses. The Scale (AGCCS) was translated into Chinese and then revised. Psychometric testing of the scale was conducted on 252 nurses who participated in the care of patients with terminal cancer at a regional teaching hospital in Southern Taiwan. The data were analyzed using descriptive statistics, reliability, and Pearson's correlation, and principal component analysis and analysis of variance were performed. Item- and scale-content validity indexes were 0.99 and 0.93, respectively. The Cronbach α of internal consistency was 0.981. The final 53-item AGCCS had five factors, which accounted for 70.81% of the total variance. The Pearson correlation coefficients of these factors ranged between 0.406 and 0.880 ($p < 0.001$). The AGCCS can be used to evaluate the aforementioned competency for improving caregivers' quality of care. It can also facilitate in-service education planning and evaluation.

Keywords: patients with terminal cancer; caregivers; competency in anticipatory grief counseling

1. Introduction

In 2021, cancer was one of the 10 leading causes of death in Taiwan, accounting for 28.0% of all deaths [1]. An integrative literature review revealed that 12.5% to 38.5% of caregivers experience anticipatory grief symptoms before the death of their relatives [2]. In caregivers of patients with terminal cancer, anticipatory grief can result in a highly stressful and conflicting experience. Nurses lack the relevant competency for assessing and managing the psychological problems encountered by these caregivers. Consequently, they are unable to address the caregivers' anticipatory grief promptly or appropriately, which in turn affects the caregivers' quality of life [3]. Inadequate assessment and management of anticipatory grief in the caregivers of patients with terminal cancer may lead to complex grief reactions [4].

In clinical nursing education, the emphasis has shifted from obtaining information using a didactic method to enhancing problem-solving through experiential learning [5]. With competency-based education, nurses are taught to fulfill the demands of the clinical care environment; moreover, competency-based assessments are applied to evaluate their competency [6]. These assessments are performed using Miller's pyramid of clinical competency and Kolb's experiential learning cycle [6].

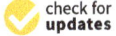

Citation: Hsiao, C.-C.; Hsieh, S.-I.; Kao, C.-Y.; Chu, T.-P. Development of a Scale of Nurses' Competency in Anticipatory Grief Counseling for Caregivers of Patients with Terminal Cancer. *Healthcare* 2023, 11, 264. https://doi.org/10.3390/healthcare11020264

Academic Editor: Margaret Fitch

Received: 15 November 2022
Revised: 10 January 2023
Accepted: 12 January 2023
Published: 14 January 2023

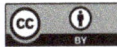

Copyright: © 2023 by the authors. Licensee MDPI, Basel, Switzerland. This article is an open access article distributed under the terms and conditions of the Creative Commons Attribution (CC BY) license (https://creativecommons.org/licenses/by/4.0/).

In Canada, hospice nurses are required to have core competencies, including assessing the needs of patients' families and providing them with knowledge on loss, grief, and bereavement. Hospice nurses must consider the stage of development and aid patients' families in recognizing the characteristics of grief and distinguishing grief and depression. The nurses must also identify family members at high risk of complex grief; assist them in predicting, recognizing, and adjusting their individual responses to loss and death; consider the unique needs of children at different developmental stages; and support the process of loss, grief, and bereavement through the grieving nursing care plan [7]. In Colombia, hospice nurses' core competencies include communication; the formation of therapeutic interpersonal relationships with patients and families; and the provision of emotional, grief, and spiritual care to these individuals [8]. The core competencies outlined by the European Association for Palliative Care include the provision of patient- and family-centered care; comfort care; psychological, social, and spiritual care; the ability to cope with ethical challenges; inter-professional cooperation; communication skills; development of interpersonal relationships with patients and families; self-awareness; and commitment to continuous professional development [9]. In Taiwan, these competencies include spiritual care, life review, and death preparation [10]. Nurses play multiple roles in grief care in terms of patient- and family-centered care, advocacy, and professional development [11–14]. They are also responsible for assessing caregivers' psychological state and providing them with emotional support by listening to them (to allow caregivers to express their emotions), and they also improve the sensitivity of grief assessment through grief counseling theory to support caregivers in managing anticipatory grief [15]. Among all healthcare providers, nurses have the most contact with patients and their families [16]. Therefore, they also have more opportunities to listen to patients (including those with terminal cancer) and caregivers and to assess their psychological distress levels. Nurses' inability to provide such care can negatively affect their patients' and caregivers' quality of life [3].

Scales for measuring anticipatory grief counseling competency, however, have been developed only in the field of counseling. The Death Counseling Survey (DCS), designed by 34 grief counseling experts, is a self-assessment of grief counselors' professional knowledge and treatment and assessment skills. It contains 58 questions scored on a 5-point Likert scale (ranging from 1 = noncompliance to 5 = full compliance). The Cronbach α of the five subscales ranges from 0.80 to 0.94. The Grief Counseling Competency Scale (GCCS) was developed by Cicchetti [17] and Cicchetti et al. [18], modified from the DCS and revised by 27 experts with >5 years of family grief counseling experience by using the Delphi method. The GCCS is a self-assessment questionnaire comprising 46 questions scored on a 5-point Likert scale (ranging from 1 = this does not describe me to 5 = this describes me very well). The questionnaire is divided into two sections comprising nine questions related to personal competency and grief and 37 questions related to skills and knowledge of grief counseling competency; the Cronbach α values of Sections 1 and 2 are 0.79 and 0.97, respectively. Of the 37 questions in the second section, questions 9, 9, and 19 address conceptual skills and knowledge, assessment skills, and treatment skills, respectively; the Cronbach α values of the three subscales in Section 2 are 0.59, 0.60, and 0.60, respectively [17].

The GCCS developed by Cicchetti [17] is primarily intended for counselors with a master's degree; it emphasizes the life experience, philosophy, and attitude toward death, diagnostic criteria of grief and its distinction from other diagnoses, use of specific death-associated words to discuss death-related matters, and ability to convey matters and explain death to children at various stages of death concept development. However, some GCCS items are unachievable for clinical nurses, and academic and in-service nurse education often lacks counseling courses. In addition, nurses are not expected to help caregivers understand the process and types of anticipatory grief, identify the manifestations of anticipatory grief, understand the differences between anticipatory grief and grief, or evaluate the risk of anticipatory grief. To the best of our knowledge, no scale has yet been developed for evaluating the competency of nurses in providing anticipatory grief counseling to caregivers of patients with terminal cancer. Therefore, in this study, we developed a scale for this purpose; psychometric testing of this scale was also conducted to evaluate the scale's content and construct validity and internal consistency reliability.

2. Materials and Methods

2.1. Design

In this psychometric study, a cross-sectional survey was conducted using a structured questionnaire, which is part of a larger survey study [19].

2.2. Participants and Setting

Participants were recruited from the oncology ward of a regional teaching hospital in southern Taiwan by using convenience sampling [20]. A sample size of 3 to 6 per item was required. The participants included nurses, nurse practitioners, case managers, and assistant head nurses who had cared for patients with terminal cancer and were 20 years or older. After sampling was completed, the study instructions and anonymous questionnaires (with codes and commodity cards) were distributed among the participants. Of the 257 questionnaires issued, 251 completed questionnaires were returned, corresponding to a response rate of 97.7%.

2.3. Instruments

The instrument developed in this study featured sociodemographic and professional background characteristics and the Anticipatory Grief Counseling Competency Scale (AGCCS). The AGCCS was adapted from the GCCS [17] and employed care provided to caregivers in hospice care in Canada for their loss, grief, and bereavement, 7 spiritual care competencies [21], and spiritual care nursing interventions [22] as references for its development. The GCCS consists of 46 items scored on a 5-point Likert scale, and the scale is divided into 2 sections, with 9 items assessing perceived personal competencies (Cronbach α = 0.79) and 37 items assessing perceived skills and knowledge competencies (Cronbach α = 0.97). The 3 subsections of the second section include 9 items on conceptual skills and knowledge (Cronbach α = 0.59), 9 items on assessment skills (Cronbach α = 0.60), and 19 items on treatment skills (Cronbach α = 0.60) [17,18]. The GCCS has been adapted from the 58-item DCS, scored on a 5-point Likert scale; it contains 5 subscales: personal competencies (Cronbach α = 0.79), conceptual skills and knowledge (Cronbach α = 0.92), assessment skills (Cronbach α = 0.63), treatment skills (Cronbach α 0.87), and professional skills (Cronbach α = 0.83) [18].

Two experts with a nursing background and doctorate who had lived in English-speaking countries for >5 years performed the English-to-Chinese translation and Chinese-to-English back translation of the questionnaires used. The initial 60 items were evaluated for content validity by a panel of 7 experts with a master's degree or higher; at least 5 years of experience in oncology, hospice, or palliative care; and who were ranked as an instructor or higher. These experts comprised 2 nursing supervisors, 1 nursing lecturer, 1 associate professor, 1 attending physician, 1 psychologist, and 1 social worker. Specifically, content validity was assessed as the topical appropriateness or relevance of the scale items on a 4-point Likert-type scale (ranging from 1 = not relevant to 4 = extremely relevant). The items were merged, added, separated, or revised according to the expert advice. After these revisions were made (55 items), a second round of expert validity review was performed, as an unfavorable scale-content validity index (S-CVI) of 0.68 was obtained. Further revision was conducted according to expert recommendations, as follows. "I can identify cultural differences in anticipatory grief care" and "I can identify cultural differences that affect responses to anticipatory grief" were combined into "I can identify cultural differences in anticipatory grief care and responses to anticipatory grief." The final questionnaire comprised 55 items, including 9 items that addressed personal experiences of anticipatory grief, self-awareness, traits, skills related to counseling, and conceptual understanding of counseling. The remaining 46 items pertained to self-evaluation of knowledge and skills related to anticipatory grief counseling and nursing. All items were scored on a 5-point Likert scale (ranging from 1 = noncompliance to 5 = full compliance).

2.4. Procedure

Figure 1 illustrates the study procedure. After permission was obtained from the author of the GCCS, forward and backward translation of the 46-item GCCS was conducted. Then, the 51-item AGCCS was developed based on cited references and through the revision of items [5,17,18]. First and second rounds of expert content validity review were conducted.

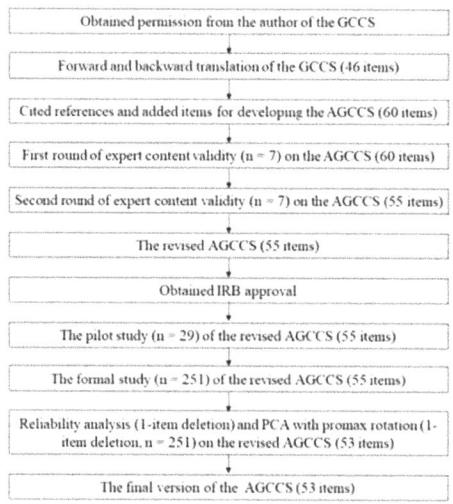

Figure 1. Study procedure.

A pilot study was conducted in the hematology, oncology, and neurosurgery departments (n = 29) between 26 November and 17 December 2019. Subsequently, the formal study was conducted in 11 units between 19 February and 6 March, 2020. Finally, the reliability and construct validity of the questionnaires were determined using the collected data.

2.5. Ethical Considerations

This study was approved by the study hospital's institutional review board (201901235B0A3). Before the questionnaire was administered, the participants were assured that they could withdraw from the study at any time without consequences to their work assessment or promotion opportunities. They were also asked to provide informed consent. Except for the subject manual, the questionnaire content was replaced by codes to protect participant anonymity.

2.6. Statistical Analysis

All statistical analyses were performed using SPSS Statistics for Windows (version 21; IBM, Armonk, NY, USA). Assumptions of normality, linearity, outliers, and multicollinearity for factor analysis were checked [23]. For sociodemographic and professional characteristics and the AGCCS scores, descriptive statistics were analyzed for frequency, percent, mean, and standard deviation. Reliability analysis was used to assess the internal consistency of the AGCCS [24]. Principal component analysis (PCA) of the exploratory factor analysis with Promax rotation was used to examine construct validity, and these analyses were based on initial eigenvalues ($\geq$1), factor loadings (>0.40), and scree plots [24,25]. Analysis of variance (ANOVA) was used to examine the mean difference in AGCCS scores on ever caring for family, relatives, and friends with anticipatory grief [26]. Pearson correlation was used to analyze the association between the AGCCS factors.

3. Results

3.1. Sociodemographic and Professional Characteristics of the Participants

Most of the participants were aged 26 to 30 years (31.1%), and nearly two-thirds were unmarried (65.3%). Moreover, 92% of the participants had a bachelor's degree in nursing, and 68.5% had religious inclinations, including 39.5% and 17% with Taoist and folk beliefs, respectively. Most (71.3%) of the participants had experiences with death, and 66.5% of the participants had experienced anticipatory grief because of the death of a relative or through relatives and friends.

Most (71.3%) of the participants were clinical nurses. The participants worked in the hematology and oncology, pulmonology, gastrointestinal and hepatobiliary pathology, or urology departments. Moreover, 36.3% and 34.3% of the participants had 5 to 10 years of experience regarding working experience in the current department and the total working years. Of all the nurses, 42.6% had taken at least one course on or received training in anticipatory grief counseling during their education (26.7%) or as a part of the in-service programs at their workplace (16.7%).

3.2. Content Validity

The item-content validity index (I-CVI) and S-CVI of the AGCCS were 0.95 and 0.68 in the first round of expert content validity evaluation, respectively, and 0.99 and 0.93 in the second round of expert content validity evaluation, respectively (Figure 1).

3.3. Construct Validity—Principal Component Analysis of the Exploratory Factor Analysis

The 55 items on the scale were subjected to PCA with Promax rotation. The value of the Kaiser–Meyer–Olkin (KMO) measure of sampling adequacy was 0.965. The measure of sampling adequacy (MSA) of individual items ranged from 0.884 to 0.987. The Bartlett test of sphericity demonstrated significance (χ^2 (1378) = 13,806.5, $p < 0.001$), with an initial eigenvalue and factor loading of >1.00 and 0.40, respectively. The items with corrected item-total correlations <0.30 (1–8, "I believe that there is more than one correct way to deal with anticipatory grief") and factor loading <0.40 (1–9, "I have a sense of humor") were excluded from the exploratory factor analysis step by step. Factors 1, 2, 3, 4, and 5 explained 52.18%, 8.08%, 5.40%, 2.67%, and 2.47% of the variance, respectively. In general, all five factors explained 70.81% of the total variance (Table 1). The scree plot in Figure 2 illustrates the five factors.

As presented in Appendix A (Table A1), the five factors of the scale were named as follows: factor 1 = competency in identification, assessment, and notification of anticipatory grief and enhancement of client's self-expression and management (19 items); factor 2 = competency in nursing interventions for anticipatory grief (13 items); factor 3 = competency in counseling for anticipatory grief (nine items); factor 4 = personal experience, self-awareness, traits, and counseling perspective and competency in addressing anticipatory grief (seven items); and factor 5 = competency in respecting, accepting, and listening to anticipatory grief and inter-professional collaboration for anticipatory grief (five items). Most of the items loaded on factors 3 and 4 between the pattern matrix and structure matrix, except two items (AGCC2-19 and AGCC2-33), were identical. The item of AGCC2-19 was loaded on factor 1 of the pattern matrix and factor 5 of the structure matrix, whereas the item of AGCC2-33 was loaded on factor 1 of the pattern matrix and factor 2 of the structure matrix.

Table 1. Total variance explained by the five factors of the Anticipatory Grief Counseling Competency Scale (n = 251).

Factor	Initial Eigenvalues			Extraction Sums of Squared Loadings		
	Total	Variance (%)	Cumulative Variance (%)	Total	Variance (%)	Cumulative Variance (%)
Factor 1: Competency in identification, assessment, and notification of anticipatory grief and enhancement of client's self-expression and management	27.66	52.18	52.18	27.66	52.18	52.18
Factor 2: Competency in nursing interventions of anticipatory grief	4.29	8.08	60.27	4.29	8.08	60.27
Factor 3: Competency in counseling of anticipatory grief	2.86	5.40	65.67	2.86	5.40	65.67
Factor 4: Personal experience, self-awareness, traits, and counseling perspective and competency in addressing anticipatory grief	1.42	2.67	68.34	1.42	2.67	68.34
Factor 5: Competency in respecting, accepting, listening to, and interprofessional collaboration for anticipatory grief	1.31	2.47	70.81	1.31	2.47	70.81

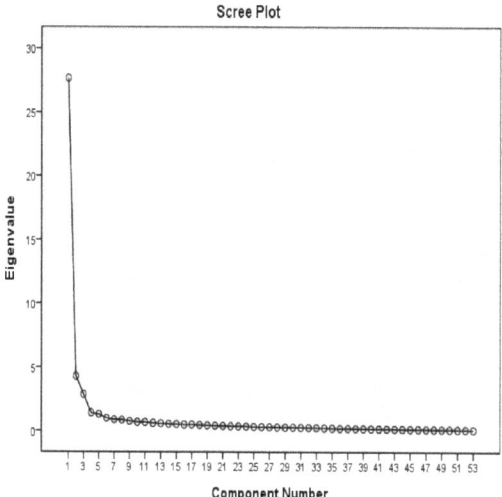

Figure 2. Scree plot.

3.4. Construct Validity—Contrasted Groups Method

Our ANOVA results revealed that the mean AGCCS scores were significantly different between the participants who had (n = 138) and those who had not (n = 113) cared for family, relatives, or friends with anticipatory grief (176.47 ± 31.54 vs. 166.19 ± 20.09, $F_{(1, 249)} = 7.07, p = 0.008$).

3.5. Internal Consistency Reliability

In the pilot study (n = 29) and the formal study, the AGCCS had a Cronbach α of 0.975. and 0.981, respectively—demonstrating its internal consistency. The items with corrected item-total correlations <0.30 (1–8, "I believe that there is more than one correct way to deal with anticipatory grief") and factor loading <0.40 (1–9, "I have a sense of humor") were excluded during the exploratory factor analysis. As presented in Table 2, the internal consistency of the five factors ranged between 0.869 and 0.974. As shown in Table 2, two-tailed Pearson's correlation revealed moderate to substantially high positive correlations between the factors ($r = 0.406$–0.880, $p < 0.01$). The correlation coefficients of factor 1 and factor 2 were the highest ($r = 0.880$, $p < 0.01$), followed by the correlation coefficients of factor 1 and factor 3 ($r = 0.820$, $p < 0.01$).

Table 2. Pearson correlation coefficients between the five factors of the Anticipatory Grief Counseling Competency Scale (n = 251).

Factor	F1	F2	F3	F4	F5
Factor 1: Competency in identification, assessment, and notification of anticipatory grief and enhancement of client's self-expression and management	1.000				
Factor 2: Competency in nursing interventions of anticipatory grief	0.880 **	1.000			
Factor 3: Competency in counseling of anticipatory grief	0.820 **	0.747 **	1.000		
Factor 4: Personal experience, self-awareness, traits, and counseling perspective and competency in addressing anticipatory grief	0.406 **	0.445 **	0.528 **	1.000	
Factor 5: Competency in respecting, accepting, listening to, and interprofessional collaboration for anticipatory grief	0.519 **	0.623 **	0.463 **	0.518 **	1.000

Note. ** $p < 0.01$ level (2-tailed).

3.6. Descriptive Statistics of the AGCCS

Table 3 presents the grand means and means of the scores for the five factors of the AGCCS, as well as their corresponding standard deviations. The grand means and standard deviations for factors 1, 2, 3, 4, and 5 were 57.10 ± 13.21, 41.05 ± 8.79, 28.90 ± 6.19, 26.84 ± 4.00, and 17.95 ± 3.29 points, respectively. The means ± standard deviations of each factor divided by the number of items ranked from high to low were as follows: factor 4: 3.83 ± 0.57, followed by the means ± standard deviations of factor 5 (3.59 ± 0.66), factor 3 (3.21 ± 0.69), factor 2 (3.16 ± 0.68), and factor 1 (3.01 ± 0.70).

Table 3. Grand means, means, and standard deviations of the five factors of the Anticipatory Grief Counseling Competency Scale (n = 251).

Factor	Grand Mean (SD)	Item	Mean (SD)
Factor 1: Competency in identification, assessment, and notification of anticipatory grief and enhancement of client's self-expression and management	57.10 (13.21)	19	3.01 (0.70)
Factor 2: Competency in nursing interventions of anticipatory grief	41.05 (8.79)	13	3.16 (0.68)
Factor 3: Competency in counseling of anticipatory grief	28.90 (6.19)	9	3.21 (0.69)
Factor 4: Personal experience, self-awareness, traits, and counseling perspective and competency in addressing anticipatory grief	26.84 (4.00)	7	3.83 (0.57)
Factor 5: Competency in respecting, accepting, listening to, and interprofessional collaboration for anticipatory grief	17.95 (3.29)	5	3.59 (0.66)

Abbreviation: SD, standard deviation.

4. Discussion

In this study, we developed and evaluated the content and validity, and internal consistency of the AGCCS for nurses. As recommended by Polit and Beck [26], the evaluation by seven experts revealed that the scale had an I-CVI and S-CVI of 0.99 and 0.93, respectively—indicating high expert content validity of individual items and the overall scale, respectively.

Rather than principal axis factoring (PAF) and PCA with promax and direct oblimin, we used PCA with promax rotation, with an oblique solution for the rotation, because most item–item correlations were >0.30. [25] The KMO measure was 0.965, and the MSA of individual items ranged between 0.884 and 0.987 (i.e., >0.60) [25]. The Bartlett test of sphericity was significant ($p < 0.001$). These values indicate sampling adequacy and initial factor extraction. The 25 Factors 1, 2, 3, 4, and 5 explained 52.18%, 8.08%, 5.40%, 2.67%, and 2.47% of the variance, respectively; moreover, all five factors explained 70.81% of the total variance. Factor 1 explained 50% more variance than the other four factors. Although factors 3, 4, and 5 explained <5% of the variance, their eigenvalues were >1. In addition, the scree plot in Figure 2 presents all five factors [25]. We also reported the pattern and structure matrices for obliquely rotated solutions and named the five factors according to their items [25].

The results of the contrasted group's method demonstrated that the mean AGCCS scores were significantly higher for the participants who had cared for family, relatives, or friends with anticipatory grief than those who had not (176.47 vs. 166.19). The contrasted group's method was used to confirm the construct validity of the AGCCS, whereby the validity was examined on the basis of the degree to which the AGCCS demonstrated different scores for the groups known to have varying AGCCS scores [26]. Nurses who have cared for family, relatives, or friends with anticipatory grief may learn how to assess, plan, manage, and evaluate anticipatory grief by reflecting and working on improving their anticipatory grief counseling competency. Real-word experience presents powerful learning opportunities by situating nurses in authentic settings relevant to their clinical roles [5]. Competency in anticipatory grief counseling varies considerably depending on whether the nurses had cared for family, relatives, or friends with anticipatory grief, but not depending on their age. These results are identical to those of Cicchetti et al. [18] and Hsieh et al. [21]. In recent years, grief-related courses have been added to the curriculum of nursing schools in Taiwan. In the past, no similar courses or anticipatory grief courses were available, which resulted in insufficient nurse willingness toward and competency in anticipatory grief counseling. Presumably, because of their own experiences with anticipatory grief, nurses became highly aware of anticipatory grief reactions and their consequences. As a result of their empathy, they became more willing to offer anticipatory grief counseling for others with identical problems. Because of their anticipatory grief experiences or self-awareness and traits, they became more likely to focus on anticipatory grief responses in patients with terminal cancer and their caregivers. Therefore, they became more aware of anticipatory grief responses and their importance. These outcomes are similar to those reported in a previous study [27].

In the pilot and formal studies, the Cronbach α of the overall scale was 0.975 and 0.981, respectively. The internal consistency reliability of the five factors ranged from 0.869 to 0.974, indicating high reliability (>0.80), and the reliability value was slightly higher than that reported by Cicchetti18 for the GCCS, and no multicollinearity was observed among the reported issues [24,26]. The high internal consistency reliability of the AGCCS may be attributable to the inclusion of more items than those included by Cicchetti [18] and because the scale specifically measures the participants' anticipatory grief counseling competency and the homogeneity among the participants in this respect [28]. This is consistent with the results of the GCCS [17,18], which was developed to measure master-level counselors involved in rehabilitation counseling. The scale was developed using the core competencies of palliative care in Canada [7] as well as spiritual care competency [21] and spiritual care nursing interventions [22] as references.

In this study, a substantially strong correlation [29] was observed between factors 1 and 2 and between factors 1 and 3. This can be explained by the fact that nurses are better able to provide anticipatory grief interventions and conduct anticipatory grief counseling when they can recognize, assess, and validate anticipatory grief and enhance clients' self-expression and management skills in nursing care. Regarding the means ± standard deviations of each factor divided by the number of items, factor 4 showed the highest mean, followed by factors 5, 3, 2, and 1. Nurses usually possessed personal experience, self-awareness, traits, counseling perspective, and competency of anticipatory grief, as well as competency in respecting, accepting, and listening to anticipatory grief and inter-professional collaboration for anticipatory grief if their workload was low. Thus, they rated factor 4 and 5 items higher than factor 1 to 3 items. The mean of factor 1 was the lowest because the participants lacked training on the identification, assessment, and notification of anticipatory grief and enhancement of clients' self-expression and management at school or in-service education. This competency can be strengthened through a series of workshops and bedside teaching methods (e.g., Objective Structured Clinical Examination and trusted professional activities based on competency) [30,31]. However, a single training session is insufficient for nurses to gain confidence in their grief counseling skills and conceptual knowledge [32].

This study has several limitations. First, this study was conducted in a single hospital, limiting the generalizability of the results. Nevertheless, the AGCCS may be used by other hospital's nurses to assess nurses' anticipatory grief counseling competency in the future and design in-service education programs. Second, the 53-item AGCCS was developed and tested in this study. Future studies can shorten it and test the construct validity of the shortened scale by using confirmatory factor analysis.

5. Conclusions

The five factors assessed for the AGCCS were significantly correlated and accounted for 70.81% of the total variance. The scale exhibited satisfactory content validity, internal consistency reliability, and construct validity. The AGCCS can be used to measure nurses' competency in anticipatory grief counseling for patients with terminal cancer, their caregivers, or patients with acute trauma, thus improving their quality of care. Therefore, the AGCCS can aid in the planning and evaluation of in-service education.

Author Contributions: Study Design, C.-C.H. and S.-I.H.; Data Collection, C.-C.H.; Data Analysis, S.-I.H.; Manuscript Preparation: C.-C.H. and S.-I.H.; Final Manuscript Approval, C.-C.H., S.-I.H., C.-Y.K. and T.-P.C. All authors have read and agreed to the published version of the manuscript.

Funding: This research was funded by the Chang Gung Memorial Research Grant of the Chang Gung Medical Foundation (CMRPG6J0311).

Institutional Review Board Statement: The study was approved by the Institutional Review Board (IRB) of a medical center in northern Taiwan (201901235B0A3, 14 October 2019).

Informed Consent Statement: Written informed consent has been obtained from all participants to publish this paper.

Data Availability Statement: The datasets used and analyzed in this study are not available be-cause of the ethics restrictions set by the IRB.

Acknowledgments: The authors would like to thank all the clinical nurses who participated in this study.

Conflicts of Interest: The authors declare no conflict of interest.

Appendix A

Table A1. Results of exploratory factor analysis using principal component analysis with Promax rotation (n = 251).

Factors and Items	Pattern Matrix	Structure Matrix	Corrected Item-Total Correlation
Factor 1: Competency in identification, assessment, and notification of anticipatory grief and enhancement of client's self-expression and management (Cronbach α = 0.974)			
2-16. I can define and explain the characteristics and symptoms of complex or unresolved anticipatory grief.	0.936	0.878	0.833
2-15. I can perform suicide risk assessment.	0.888	0.762	0.721
2-13. I can lead a consultation meeting on anticipatory grief.	0.815	0.841	0.798
2-23. I can provide appropriate crisis interview, records, and briefings.	0.775	0.848	0.828
2-17. I can teach the individual to obtain community support and resources for managing anticipatory grief.	0.768	0.842	0.820
2-18. I can assess the state of the individual's spiritual well-being (peaceful mood).	0.698	0.833	0.828
2-14. I can describe individual differences in anticipatory grief.	0.678	0.849	0.833
2-11. I can identify individuals at risk of complex anticipatory grief.	0.675	0.841	0.825
2-21. I can identify cultural differences in care for and response to anticipatory grief.	0.672	0.814	0.824
2-27. I can describe a typical dysfunctional coping style of an individual experiencing anticipatory grief.	0.666	0.872	0.875
2-22. I can use family assessment techniques to examine the interaction patterns and roles among family members.	0.662	0.820	0.822
2-26. I can improve the individual's ability to handle their anticipatory grief response.	0.655	0.831	0.834
2-19. I can build a trusting relationship with individuals of all ages.	0.647	0.627	0.614
2-10. I can differentiate between the characteristics of anticipatory grief and depression.	0.614	0.801	0.793
2-12. I can conduct personal anticipatory grief consultations.	0.605	0.837	0.831
2-28. I can assess the progress of the individual's anticipatory grief.	0.547	0.848	0.859
2-29. I can use creative or artistic media to guide the individual to express anticipatory grief.	0.519	0.806	0.800
2-33. I can identify and deal with resistance and denial related to anticipatory grief.	0.468	0.745	0.754
2-34. I can describe effective responses to anticipatory grief.	0.468	0.789	0.798
Factor 2: Competency in nursing interventions of anticipatory grief (Cronbach α = 0.958)			
2-35. I can participate in informal or formal support groups organized by anticipatory grief professionals to prevent burnout and cope with the trauma resulting from witnessing suffering.	0.813	0.775	0.651
2-37. I can recommend helpful articles and books on anticipatory grief for individuals or families.	0.762	0.818	0.714
2-43. I can provide care to individuals experiencing anticipatory grief.	0.743	0.875	0.776
2-42. I incorporate anticipatory grief care into my nursing plans.	0.732	0.837	0.857
2-44. I can assess effectiveness of the anticipatory grief care provided by myself or my team.	0.716	0.879	0.813
2-31. I constantly update the anticipatory grief-related resources to my clients.	0.678	0.795	0.867

Table A1. Cont.

Factors and Items	Pattern Matrix	Structure Matrix	Corrected Item-Total Correlation
2-36. I can apply various counseling theories to individual and family counseling for anticipatory grief.	0.667	0.815	0.781
2-40. I can revise the care plan for a client according to their needs or problems related to anticipatory grief.	0.640	0.806	0.800
2-41. I can revise care plans through consultation with my team members.	0.633	0.800	0.776
2-45. Peer discussion helps me identify issues related to anticipatory grief care.	0.626	0.739	0.774
2-46. I can guide others in providing anticipatory grief care.	0.570	0.826	0.691
2-30. I can share my own experience of anticipatory grief.	0.497	0.722	0.830
2-25. I stay abreast of the latest research on anticipatory grief and its effective management and apply relevant skills to my work.	0.420	0.747	0.710
Factor 3: Competency in counseling of anticipatory grief (Cronbach α = 0.953)			
2-6. I can convene family consultation meetings on anticipatory grief.	0.861	0.888	0.847
2-7. I can help individual family members predict and adjust their anticipatory grief responses.	0.855	0.910	0.885
2-2. I can identify anticipatory grief in an individual who does not show any obvious signs of it as well as assess unresolved anticipatory grief.	0.816	0.829	0.776
2-4. I can provide psychological guidance for an individual experiencing anticipatory grief.	0.787	0.875	0.847
2-3. I can provide information about anticipatory grief.	0.751	0.833	0.802
2-5. I can help families understand the concept and process of anticipatory grief and provide referrals as necessary.	0.712	0.825	0.791
2-1. I can perform an anticipatory grief needs assessment.	0.603	0.777	0.743
2-8. I can help my patients' families understand their anticipatory grief response and use a care plan to help them through the process.	0.601	0.846	0.837
2-9. I can explain and differentiate between the characteristics of "common" anticipatory grief using theoretical models	0.522	0.792	0.766
Factor 4: Personal experience, self-awareness, traits, and counseling perspective and competency in adressing anticipatory grief (Cronbach α = 0.893)			
1-2. I can verbally express my own anticipatory grief process.	0.904	0.815	0.708
1-3. I am aware of my own anticipatory grief experience and process.	0.891	0.828	0.729
1-4. I believe that anticipatory grief is linked to death and other experiences of loss.	0.790	0.782	0.694
1-6. I regard anticipatory grief as a systematic and personal experience of the body, mind, and spirit.	0.752	0.805	0.741
1-1. I take care of my own health and practice self-care.	0.728	0.767	0.679
1-7. My spiritual experience is crucial to my understanding of anticipatory grief.	0.702	0.757	0.668
1-5. I can show empathy, sincerity, and unconditional support or care toward my friends and acquaintances.	0.526	0.691	0.625

Table A1. *Cont.*

Factors and Items	Pattern Matrix	Structure Matrix	Corrected Item-Total Correlation
Factor 5: Competency in respecting, accepting, listening to, and interprofessional collaboration for anticipatory grief (Cronbach α = 0.869)			
2-32. I can provide care to the clients without prejudice, regardless of their spiritual or religious beliefs.	0.830	0.781	0.674
2-20. I can work in and interact with members of an interdisciplinary team.	0.723	0.788	0.637
2-39. I treat my clients with sympathy, empathy, sincerity, sensitivity, and respect and inspire trust in them.	0.710	0.816	0.734
2-24. I have effective active listening skills.	0.707	0.778	0.697
2-38. I can listen to the clients and allow them to share their feelings and experiences of anticipatory grief without judgment.	0.557	0.756	0.727

Note. factor > 0.4.

References

1. Ministry of Health and Welfare. The Statistical Results of National Ten Leading Causes of Death in 2021. Available online: https://www.mohw.gov.tw/cp-16-70314-1.html. (accessed on 25 September 2022).
2. Coelho, A.; Barbosa, A. Family Anticipatory Grief: An Integrative Literature Review. *Am. J. Hosp. Palliat. Med.* **2017**, *34*, 774–785. [CrossRef] [PubMed]
3. Matthews, H.; Grunfeld, E.A.; Turner, A. The Efficacy of Interventions to Improve Psychosocial Outcomes Following Surgical Treatment for Breast Cancer: A Systematic Review and Meta-analysis. *Psycho-Oncol.* **2017**, *26*, 593–607. [CrossRef] [PubMed]
4. Nielsen, M.K.; Neergaard, M.A.; Jensen, A.B.; Bro, F.; Guldin, M.B. Do We Need to Change Our Understanding of Anticipatory Grief in Caregivers? A Systematic Review of Caregiver Studies during End-of-life Caregiving and Bereavement. *Clin. Psychol. Rev.* **2016**, *44*, 75–93. [CrossRef] [PubMed]
5. Cahn, P.S.; Smoller, S.L. Experiential Learning and Cultural Competence: What Do Participants in Short-term Experiences in Global Health Learn about Culture? *Health Prof. Educ.* **2020**, *6*, 230–237. [CrossRef]
6. Jacob, S.A.; Power, A.; Portlock, J.; Jebara, T.; Cunningham, S.; Boyter, A.C. Competency-based Assessment in Experiential Learning in Undergraduate Pharmacy Programmes: Qualitative Exploration of Facilitators' Views and Needs (ACTp study). *Pharmacy.* **2022**, *10*, 90. [CrossRef] [PubMed]
7. Grantham, D.; O'Brien, L.A.; Widger, K.; Bouvette, M.; McQuinn, P. Nursing Competencies Case Examples. *Canadian Hosp. Palliat. Care.* **2009**, 1–52. Available online: https://www.virtualhospice.ca/Assets/Canadian%20Hospice%20Palliative%20Care%20Nursing%20Competencies%27%20Case%20Examples_20091208122014.pdf (accessed on 13 January 2023).
8. Pastrana, T.; Wenk, R.; De Lima, L. Consensus-based Palliative Care Competencies for Undergraduate Nurses and Physicians: A Demonstrative Process with Colombian Universities. *J. Palliat. Med.* **2016**, *19*, 76–82. [CrossRef]
9. Gamondi, C.; Larkin, P.; Payne, S. Core Competencies in Palliative Care: An EAPC White Paper on Palliative Care Education: Part 1. *Eur. J. Palliat. Care* **2013**, *20*, 86–91.
10. Hu, W.Y.; Yeh, M.C. The Perspectives on Palliative Nursing Education. *J. Nurs.* **2015**, *62*, 25–33. [CrossRef]
11. Chan, H.Y.; Lee, L.H.; Chan, C.W. The Perceptions and Experiences of Nurses and Bereaved Families towards Bereavement Care in an Oncology Unit. *Support. Care Cancer* **2013**, *21*, 1551–1556. [CrossRef]
12. Kurian, M.J.; Daniel, S.; James, A.; James, C.; Joseph, L.; Malecha, A.T.; Martin, E.M.; Mick, J.M. Intensive Care Registered Nurses' Role in Bereavement Support. *J. Hosp. Palliat. Nurs.* **2014**, *16*, 31–39. [CrossRef]
13. Mak, Y.W.; Lim Chiang, V.C.; Chui, W.T. Experiences and Perceptions of Nurses Caring for Dying Patients and Families in the Acute Medical Admission Setting. *Int. J. Palliat. Nurs.* **2013**, *19*, 423–431. [CrossRef] [PubMed]
14. Raymond, A.; Lee, S.F.; Bloomer, M.J. Understanding the Bereavement Care Roles of Nurses within Acute Care: A Systematic Review. *J. Clin. Nurs.* **2017**, *26*, 1787–1800. [CrossRef]
15. Shore, J.C.; Gelber, M.W.; Koch, L.M.; Sower, E. Anticipatory Grief: An Evidence-based Approach. *J. Hosp. Palliat. Nurs.* **2016**, *18*, 15–19. [CrossRef]
16. Budden, L.M.; Hayes, B.A.; Buettner, P.G. Women's Decision Satisfaction and Psychological Distress Following Early Breast Cancer Treatment: A Treatment Decision Support Role for Nurses. *Int. J. Nurs. Pract.* **2014**, *20*, 8–16. [CrossRef] [PubMed]
17. Cicchetti, R.J. Graduate Students' Self Assessment of Competency in Grief Education and Training in Core Accredited Rehabilitation Counseling Programs. Ph.D. Thesis, Old Dominion University, Norfolk, VA, USA, 2010.
18. Cicchetti, R.J.; McArthur, L.; Szirony, G.M.; Blum, C. Perceived Competency in Grief Counseling: Implications for Counselor Education. *J. Soc. Behav. Health Sci.* **2016**, *10*, 2. [CrossRef]
19. Hsiao, C.C.; Hsieh, S.I.; Kao, C.Y.; Chu, T.P. Factors Affecting Nurses' Willingness and Competency to Provide Anticipatory Grief Counseling for Family Caregivers of Patients with Terminal Cancer. *J. Clin. Nurs.* **2022**, *32*. [CrossRef]
20. De Winter, J.C.F.; Dodou, D.; Wieringa, P.A. Exploratory Factor Analysis with Small Sample Sizes. *Multivar. Behav. Res.* **2009**, *44*, 147–181. [CrossRef] [PubMed]
21. Hsieh, S.I.; Hsu, L.L.; Kao, C.Y.; Breckenridge-Sproat, S.; Lin, H.L.; Tai, H.C.; Huang, T.H.; Chu, T.L. Factors Associated with Spiritual Care Competencies in Taiwan's Clinical Nurses: A Descriptive Correlational Study. *J. Clin. Nurs.* **2020**, *29*, 1599–1613. [CrossRef]
22. Caldeira, S.I.; Timmins, F. Implementing Spiritual Care Interventions. *Nurs. Stand.* **2017**, *31*, 54–60. [CrossRef]
23. Tabachnick, B.G.; Fidell, L.S. Principal Components and Factor Analysis. In *Using Multivariate Statistics*, 5th ed.; Pearson Education: Boston, MA, USA, 2007; pp. 607–675.
24. Field, A. Exploratory Factor Analysis. In *Discovering Satistics Using IBM SPSS Statistics*, 5th ed.; Sage: Brighton, UK, 2018; pp. 627–685.
25. Pett, M.A.; Lackey, N.R.; Sullivan, J.J. *Making Sense of Factor Analysis: The Use of Factor Analysis for Instrument Development in Health Care Research*; Sage: New York, NY, USA, 2003.
26. Polit, D.F.; Beck, C.T. *Nursing Research: Generating and Assessing Evidence for Nursing Practice*, 11th ed.; Wolters Kluwer: Alphen aan den Rijn, The Netherlands, 2021.
27. Wheat, L.S.; Matthews, J.J.; Whiting, P.P. Grief Content Inclusion in CACREP-Accredited Counselor Education Programs. *J. Couns. Prep. Superv.* **2022**, *15*, 14.
28. Waltz, C.F.; Strickland, O.L.; Lenz, E.R. *Measurement in Nursing and Health Research*, 3rd ed.; Springer: Berlin/Heidelberg, Germany, 2005; pp. 137–153.

29. Akoglu, H. User's Guide to Correlation Coefficients. *Turk. J. Emerg. Med.* **2018**, *18*, 91–93. [CrossRef] [PubMed]
30. Khan, K.Z.; Ramachandran, S.; Gaunt, K.; Pushkar, P. The Objective Structured Clinical Examination (OSCE): AMEE Guide No. 81. Part I: An Historical and Theoretical Perspective. *Med. Teach.* **2013**, *35*, e1437–e1446. [CrossRef] [PubMed]
31. Association of American Medical Colleges. The Core Entrustable Professional Activities (EPAs) for Entering Residency. Available online: https://www.aamc.org/about-us/mission-areas/medical-education/cbme/core-epas (accessed on 9 January 2023).
32. Linich, K.P. The Effects of Holistic Grief Counseling Training on. Master's Level Counseling Students' Grief and Loss Counseling Competency. Ph.D. Dissertation, South Carolina University, Columbia, SC, USA, 2021.

Disclaimer/Publisher's Note: The statements, opinions and data contained in all publications are solely those of the individual author(s) and contributor(s) and not of MDPI and/or the editor(s). MDPI and/or the editor(s) disclaim responsibility for any injury to people or property resulting from any ideas, methods, instructions or products referred to in the content.

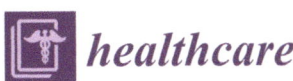

Article

Do You Feel Safe at Home? A Qualitative Study among Home-Dwelling Older Adults with Advanced Incurable Cancer

Ellen Karine Grov [1,*,†] and Siri Ytrehus [2,†]

1. Department of Nursing and Health Promotion, Faculty of Health Sciences, Oslo Metropolitan University, 0130 Oslo, Norway
2. Department of Health and Caring Sciences, Western University of Applied Sciences, 5020 Bergen, Norway
* Correspondence: ellgro@oslomet.no; Tel.: +47-6723-6378
† These authors contributed equally to this work.

Abstract: Many older adults with cancer prefer to live at home, and home treatment and outpatient care have been recommended for such patients. To improve their mental health, it is important to identify the challenges that are faced by home-dwelling older adults with cancer. This study aimed to examine the impact of the home on older adults with advanced cancer who were receiving treatment and follow-up care. In a cross-sectional design with criterion-based sampling, eight qualitative interviews were transcribed and interpreted thematically. We identified three themes of home-safety management: good home-safety management, uncertain home-safety management, and home-safety management collapse. Moreover, we revealed eight sub-themes important to the participants' home-safety experience. Ensuring that older adults feel safe at home will afford them the opportunity to enjoy living at home, which in turn may alleviate their symptom burden and enhance their mental health.

Keywords: cancer care; older adults; mental health; feeling safe; home-dwelling

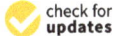

Citation: Grov, E.K.; Ytrehus, S. Do You Feel Safe at Home? A Qualitative Study among Home-Dwelling Older Adults with Advanced Incurable Cancer. *Healthcare* **2022**, *10*, 2384. https://doi.org/10.3390/healthcare10122384

Academic Editor: Paolo Cotogni

Received: 25 October 2022
Accepted: 20 November 2022
Published: 28 November 2022

Publisher's Note: MDPI stays neutral with regard to jurisdictional claims in published maps and institutional affiliations.

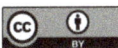

Copyright: © 2022 by the authors. Licensee MDPI, Basel, Switzerland. This article is an open access article distributed under the terms and conditions of the Creative Commons Attribution (CC BY) license (https://creativecommons.org/licenses/by/4.0/).

1. Introduction

As the World Health Organization states, mental health " ... goes beyond the mere absence of a mental health condition" and includes, e.g., social, cultural, and other interrelated factors contributing to mental health [1]. With this broad definition, we assume safety and reduced risk of harm as aspects of mental health on both system and individual levels. Thus, with support from a Finnish study, we argue that mental well-being and dwelling in a safe environment are linked together [2]. Over the past few decades, health authorities have underscored the role that the home plays in the lives of older adults with advanced health problems and the need for home care and social services [3–6]. The relationships that older adults share with their homes and communities have been gaining renewed research attention as a result of the increase in the number of older adults and the commonness of a combination of out-patient treatment services and home-based care and treatment. Many older adults continue to live in their own homes even when they have advanced cancer, receive advanced treatment, and follow-up palliative care [7–9].

Currently, in many countries, health care service providers assume that home-based care is more cost effective than institutional care [10], and it is assumed that older adults wish to continue living in their homes for as long as possible [11]. However, some of these assumptions have been questioned [11,12].

1.1. The Meaning of a Home to Older Adults

Across the fields of social geography, sociology, and gerontology, the dominating perspective on homes is that the home should be understood not only as a physical space within which various events take place but also as an entity that is influenced by both emotional, mental, and social factors [13,14]. Different conceptualisations of a home have been documented in the literature [13]. Research studies on older adults and their homes have focused on the meaning that older adults ascribe to the physical, emotional, mental, and social dimensions of a home. The importance of the social and emotional dimensions of a home have been repeatedly underscored, and safety, which is one aspect of these dimensions, has been regarded as a central component of attachment between a person and his or her home [15]. The feeling of safety that a home engenders is emphasised as a fundamental sense of safety or ontological security that is embedded within the material surroundings [16].

1.2. The Home and Older Adults with Cancer

Relatively little is known about the assistance that older adults with cancer need [17–19], their experience of having advanced incurable cancer while living at home [20], and the effects of treatment on their mental and social functioning [21,22]. Similarly, little is known about the meanings that home-dwelling older adults with advanced cancer assign to a home whilst living alone. It can be very difficult to live alone under such circumstances [9,17,19,23]. Older adults are likely to be dependent on others (who often do not belong to the household) for all of their activities. Living alone can exacerbate their sense of uncertainty about the future [23,24]. Older adults with cancer who live in rural areas are a particularly vulnerable group [19,25–27]. Long distances to hospitals can limit their access to requisite help [28,29]. Furthermore, they have to travel afar to gain access to treatment services and health institutions. Norwegian studies, which were conducted among home-dwelling older adults with cancer in rural areas, found that older adults consider waiting for transportation and uncomfortable post-treatment transportation to their homes to be sources of great distress [19,25].

Palliative care research has focused on the therapeutic role that close physical surroundings in in-patient settings play during this final phase of life [30,31]. Palliative care research studies have shown that older adults prefer to die in their own homes [30,32,33]. However, this contention has been challenged because the pertinent studies have not adequately accounted for the alternatives that are available to them. There have only been a few attempts to examine safety initiatives within the home care sector [34,35]. Within a patient's home, his or her safety is inextricably linked to that of his or her carer [34]. Trusting staff, being comfortable and well informed, and engaging in daily life activities contribute to well-being and a sense of security among those who receive palliative home care [35,36]. However, there is a lack of research findings on the dimensions of a home that contribute to a sense of safety.

Therefore, this study aimed to identify the dimensions of a home that older adults consider to be important and examine the role that advanced cancer plays in the meanings that older adults with this disease assign to their homes and their feelings of safety and mental well-being when living at home. The resultant findings can be used to develop strategies that promote the safety of home-dwelling older adults with serious health problems and accommodate their extensive needs for assistance. We have outlined the following questions for this study: what role does the home play for the older adults living at home with an advanced cancer disease, what role does the disease play in the meaning of the home, and which dimensions of the home are highlighted as significant?

2. Methodology

Qualitative research methods facilitate the identification of the nuances of the relationships that individuals share with spaces [37,38]. Therefore, a qualitative cross-sectional research design was adopted in this study with criterion sampling, and we found thematic analysis suitable for data navigation [39].

2.1. Recruitment Strategy and Sample

In this study, participants were recruited in collaboration with nurses in the home care service representing four municipalities. Older adults who met the inclusion criteria received documents that (a) requested their participation in the study, (b) provided information about the study, and (c) required them to provide informed consent. Their responses to the request were relayed to the researcher. Men and women who were older than 60 years and had advanced incurable cancer were eligible for inclusion. The exclusion criteria were as follows: individuals with a cognitive impairment or a condition (e.g., terminally ill patients) that interferes with their ability to participate in an interview. A total of eight older adults from the four municipalities agreed to participate in this study. This study comprises of municipalities with 10,000–25,000 inhabitants, defined by us as rural or sub-urban.

The ages of the participants ranged from 60 to 86 years (Table 1). Five of them were men, and three of them were women. Three of them lived alone, and the others lived with a partner or spouse. They all lived in their own private homes. The participants had the following different types of cancer: breast, colorectal, prostate, bladder, oesophageal, and oesophageal and tracheal cancer. One participant had more than one type of cancer. All participants demonstrated poor functioning and had major health problems, which were caused by cancer, but the consequences of cancer and health problems varied across participants. We had no access to the participants' medical or nursing record. With these limitations, we have no objective assessment as Karnofsky or ECOG performance status. Thus, we have described their health conditions in the same way that they told us and based on our assessment. Both authors have practiced as nurses for several decades. All the participants received public or private assistance.

Table 1. Description of participants by gender, age, living arrangements, disease and health issues, public health services, and help from family/partner.

Gender, Age, Living Arrangements	Disease/Function/ Health Issues	Assistance	Help from Partner/Family
A. Male, 74 years old, lives with wife.	Lung cancer with metastasis to colon. Leakage from colon following surgery. Breathing problems and poor mobility due to hip problems. Was able to go out to his own car until a few months ago. Can barely walk up and down stairs. Previous heart attack and thrombosis. Uses several medicines.	Private home services.	Son helps with shopping.
B. Male, 78 years old, lives alone.	Prostate cancer with metastasis to bones. Chemotherapy, no curative intention. Out-patient treatment. Very weak during weekly chemotherapy. Severe pain and uses morphine-based pain relief plasters. Weak and tired, sleeps poorly, and anxiety issues. Confusion, but he attributes this to sleep medication. COPD. Has venous access port (VAP), and urinary catheter.	Receives treatment from various hospitals: national cancer hospital, central hospital, and local hospital. Some private home health services.	Some help from neighbours.
C. Male, 82 years old, lives with wife.	Bone marrow cancer, back fracture, operated to stabilise joints. In a lot of pain, reduced vision, and swollen legs. Chemotherapy and morphine-based plasters. Eating problems. Needs help to get out of bed and help to move around.	Home care nurse assists with medication administration.	Wife helps moving around indoors.
D. Female, 60 years old, lives with husband.	Breast cancer with pelvic and head metastasis. Somewhat disoriented due to the metastasis to the head. Coordination problems. Weight loss during treatment. Previous hip fracture still bothering her. Unable to go out on her own.	Home care nurse. Days in a palliative unit. Followed up by primary physician.	Husband helps with all practical tasks at home. He also helps his wife moving indoors and outdoors.

Table 1. Cont.

Gender, Age, Living Arrangements	Disease/Function/ Health Issues	Assistance	Help from Partner/Family
E. Female, 71 years old, lives with partner.	Oesophageal and tracheal cancer, heavy breathing, heart problems, diabetes, and several wounds. Enteral nutrition only. Difficulties walking stairs. Unable to go out on her own. Difficulties sleeping, prescribed sleeping pills.	Help from home care nurse several times a week. Follow-up by primary physician.	Husband deals with enteral nutrition and administration of medication.
F. Female, 68 years old, lives with her husband.	Breast cancer and colorectal cancer with colostomy. Special diet, significant weight loss. Tired and weak, becomes dizzy, and balance issues. Difficulties sleeping. Still receiving chemotherapy as tablets. Changes bandages every day. Can go out on her own.	Colostomy nurse weekly.	Husband helps with all practical tasks at home.
G. Male, 80 years old, lives alone, son has apartment in same house.	Cancer of the bladder, urostomy, diabetes, and all toes on one leg amputated. Has received radiation treatment. In a lot of pain. Physical therapy. Goes out on his own.	Home care nurse daily. Needs help with caring for fistula, administration of medication, and showering.	
H. Male, 86 years, lives alone old, partner stops by occasionally.	Prostate cancer, in wheel-chair. Has stair lift and many aids installed in home. Impaired mobility, but the kitchen is well modified and he has a telephone on a table right next to where the wheelchair is placed.	Home care nurse daily. Needs help with showering and shopping	No help from family, but partner stops by occasionally. Considered moving.

2.2. Interviews

A semi-structured interview guide that covered specific topics, which were identified from the literature, was developed. The interviews were conducted in the participants' homes. The participants reported that they felt relaxed during the interview, and they were given the opportunity to show us their homes. In the first interview, both authors served as active interviewers. The intention was to harmonise the way the interviews were conducted, and the data were collected. Regarding the other interviews, the first and last author conducted four and three interviews, respectively. The interviews were conducted with the assistance of the interview guide. The following are a few sample questions: can you describe what it is like to live at home when you have cancer? What does being able to live at home mean to you? What kind of help do you receive, and what are your experiences of receiving such help? Follow-up questions were used to facilitate further reflection upon and exploration of participants' experiences. Such questions were: how do you deal with daily activities at home? Do you find any tasks challenging? Please tell about making meals. Follow-up questions on shopping and cooking were conducted. What does this house mean to you? Please describe what is preferable, if so, of staying at home despite your serious illness. Are you able to walk outdoors? Do you need help from others to make the bed and clean the house? Who are your helpers? Are you receiving support or help from the home care nursing service?

Each interview lasted for 70 to 120 min. The spouses or partners of the participants participated in four interviews. They participated because the older adults wanted them to.

All the interviews were recorded and transcribed. The names and locations of the participants were deidentified during transcription. In this article, we present parts of the interviews, where 'I' refers to the interviewer and A-H are letters representing the patients' voice. We have connected the letters A-H to the quotations, a system that corresponds to the tables.

2.3. Analysis

Thematic analysis was used [39] whereby the data were analysed from quotations through sub-themes and themes ending with an overarching theme. Firstly, we became familiar with the data, a process which had already started while interviewing the participants. We separately read the transcripts and the noted text parts (coding units) and then in face-to-face meetings, we discussed our understanding of what we interpreted as the essential meaning. The authors always had the research questions in mind (the home's role for the patient, and the disease's impact on the meaning of the home). No software was used for the thematic analysis, as the authors wanted to read the text several times and wanted closeness to the data. From the text parts (coding unites), we identified central quotations and from these, we suggested and discussed sub-themes, themes, and the overarching theme. In the dialogue, we viewed the overarching theme, the themes and the sub-themes the other way—by turning back to the quotations. In Table 2, we present descriptions of 'good home-safety management'; 'uncertain home-safety management' and 'home-safety management collapse'. Each of the sub-themes have connected quotations in the text and we have used headings corresponding to the sub-themes and themes in the Results session.

Table 2. The overarching theme 'home-safe management' with themes and sub-themes.

	Home-Safety Management	
Good Home-Safety Management	**Uncertain Home-Safety Management**	**Home-Safety Management Collapse**
Valuable characteristics of the homes—predictability and house quality Caregiver availability and close relationship Activities, memories, and independent life in the home	Independent but unprotected Feeling insecure about living at home	Spending part of the days alone in the home High symptom burden Unable to move around

However, we have exceeded the analysis to show our interpretation of each of the participants' positions on home-safety management. In Table 3, we provide a schematic overview of our analysis presented in four phases. In phase 1, we systematically examined and reviewed the transcripts and coded the data by critically analysing the text. We found descriptions of the home as a point of departure, where the dimension of the home included the environment, the house and the role that cancer played in the participants' lives as well as the life situation with the availability of a partner, family or neighbours.

In phase 2, we shed light on what impacts each participant experienced, and a person-centred perspective from the participants (A–H) and contextual analysis [38] was conducted to examine the significance of various dimensions of the home in relation to each participant's overall life situation. In this analytic phase, we directed our attention towards the sub-themes (referred in Table 3) that had emerged from the interview data of each participant. The aspects of the participants' life situations were embedded within the interview data, and we therefore classified this phase with dimensions of the participants' life situation. Phase 3 focuses on the analytical approach, which allowed us to understand the meanings that the older adults with advanced cancer ascribed to a home. The disease is present for the participants, and we have labelled this phase 'the disease's role in the meaning of the home'. In phase 4, the themes of home-safety management were described, and the characteristics of the participants' home-safety management were identified. The matrix presented in Table 3 summarises the phases of this analytical process.

2.4. Ethics

The Regional Committees for Medical and Health Research Ethics (no.1524) and the chief health officer in each municipality approved this study. The data were stored in a secure location during the study and will be moved to the Norwegian Sikt (https://sikt.no/) (accessed on 24 October 2022).

Table 3. Schematic overview of analysis phases and the characteristics of the participants and their connected home-safety management.

	Phase 1	Phase 2	Phase 3	Phase 4
	Home dimension	Dimensions of the participant's life situation	The disease's role in the meaning of the home	Characteristics of home-safety management
Participant: A C E	Possibilities for going outdoors on the terrace and the balcony. spaciousness, takes pride in the home. Lives with partner.	The disease affects daily life to a great extent. Partner's contribution is extensive. The partner's contribution is both explicit and implicit. Emphasises meaningful and valued qualities of the home.	Enjoys the home. The disease underscores the meaning of the home. At the same time, the home places the disease in the background.	Good home-safety management. Home-safety management partly coped with by the participant or taken over by caregivers or relatives.
Participant: B	Activities, memories, interior, takes pride in the home. Lives alone.	The disease affects daily life to a great extent. Makes great personal efforts to remain in the home. Emphasises own efforts in forming the home.	Enjoys the home. The disease underscores the meaning of the home. At the same time, the home places the disease in the background.	Good home-safety management. Independent safety management.
Participant: F H	Takes pride in the home, garden, terrace, emotional attachment to the home, wants independence. One lives alone, one with a partner.	The disease necessitates extra efforts to remain in the home, but everyday life is, in the main, the same as before. Emphasises meaningful and valuable qualities of the home and own efforts in forming the home.	Enjoys the home. Considers moving but is uncertain. The disease creates uncertainty regarding the home in the future.	Uncertain home-safety management.
Participant: D G	Emphasises no aspect of the home. Lives with partner/family.	The disease affects daily life to a great extent. The participant is passive and immobile, cannot go out without help, difficulties moving around, has periodically not received needed help.	Does not wish to be alone in the home. Expresses no enjoyment of the home. The disease makes the participants unable to enjoy the home.	Home-safety management collapse.

Data services and storage (giving data access in the Norwegian language) will be conducted after the completion of the study. The participants provided informed consent, and they were informed about their right to withdraw from the study at any time.

3. Results

3.1. Good Home-Safety Management

This theme comprises of the informants' descriptions on their wish to stay at home and their feeling of being safe at home. Several participants wanted to continue living in their own homes, despite their extensive health issues and uncertainty about the progress of their disease. They wished to maintain the home as it was and reported that they thrived when they were at home and experienced well-being there.

3.2. Valuable Characteristics of the Homes—Predictability and House Quality

The health issues of some participants made them particularly aware of the value of their home. Two male participants expressed their gratitude for being able to continue living in their homes. The disease had forced them to give up engaging in a variety of activities. They reported that their homes afforded them the opportunity to spend time outdoors. One of them emphasised the satisfaction, mental well-being, and pride that he derived from living in a single-family dwelling and being able to walk in the garden that surrounded his house. He reported that this was something that he did not take for granted, given his high age and his advanced disease.

C: Well, yes, that's how it is. We're lucky to be alive; we're the oldest people around here, more or less. Oh, we are just so grateful for this!

I: Yes.

C: We're really doing fine. We can walk outdoors, you know.

One of the other participants in this theme had advanced metastatic cancer and needed assistance with most daily tasks, including mobility. The disease prevented him from travelling or going for walks. The activities that he engaged in in his home were a positive compensation for the activities that he had to give up.

A: We have not gone any further than the terrace and the deck. But it's amazing how great that can be too.

I: Yes.

A: We've said a few times, this summer, that this hotel here is certainly a pretty good place to live.

3.3. Caregiver Availability and Close Relationship

Both these men lived with a partner who played a central role in their current lives. The partners actively participated in the interviews. The men emphasised that their female partners had taken on substantial and necessary responsibilities for their care. Both stated that they would not have been able to live at home without their partners. They both said that they felt safe and wanted to continue living in their current home.

One of the female participants (E) expressed a strong desire to continue living in her home. Her partner also participated in the interview. She lived in an old apartment building that was located at the centre of a mid-size municipality. Her living conditions were significantly poorer than those of the other participants. It was difficult to access the apartment because it had a steep staircase. She had to exit the apartment to use the bathroom and toilet. Nevertheless, she strongly emphasised that she wished to continue living in her home. The municipality had offered her a new and better-adapted house in an assisted living facility. She and her partner had declined this offer. Her partner was better informed about the disease and treatment than she was. Indeed, he reported that he was responsible for contacting the health services and he was involved in performing other household tasks. However, his contributions were different from those of the other partners. Specifically, neither he nor the woman explicitly emphasised that his contribution played a decisive role in her ability to continue living in her home. The participant repeated several times during the interview that she was independent.

E: "I want to stay here. He wants to stay here. This is our home!"

3.4. Activities, Memories, and Independent Life in the Home

A third male participant in this theme of good home-safety management had advanced prostate cancer. He lived alone in a single-family dwelling with a garden in a rural area. He had always lived alone. He faced many challenges as a result of his cancer. He reported a series of problems, such as the following, for which it had been difficult to receive help: pain, problems with mobility, incontinence, and uncertainties about changes in and the progress of the disease. Nevertheless, he emphasised that he thrived, felt safe at home, and was able to make his own decisions. Furthermore, he was surrounded by familiar objects and lived in an environment that he had a part in creating. He also spoke about his interest in interior design.

I: You have said a bit about wanting to live at home. What does that mean to you?

B: Quite a lot.

I: Could you say a bit more about this? In which way?

B: I feel good here.
I: What is it that makes you feel good here?
B: My surroundings—they're just what I want.
I: How's that?
B: Furniture, curtains. I sew it all myself. I sew curtains for people too.

He wished to continue living in his home. His stories about his exhausting treatment journeys made it apparent that he had taken great efforts to continue living in his home.

B: What was exhausting was the bus drive with the Health Express from X (located far away from the specialist hospital) and down to XX (specialist hospital) and back. It took six hours.
I: Yes.
B: It was exhausting, but I had to get home to my own bed and my cat.

3.5. Uncertain Home-Safety Management

In this theme, we revealed a lot of uncertainty. This was expressed in terms of concerns about the home being the right dwelling place and the feeling of being insecure at home and uncertainty about the future because of the disease's progression. In some individuals, the disease created a sense of uncertainty about whether they ought to move. This was the case for participants who lived alone in single-family dwellings. They did not know what sort of assistance they would need in the future and how the disease would progress; therefore, they considered moving. However, both participants expressed that they felt safe at home at the time of the interview. Thus, they had considered moving because the disease had created uncertainty about the future, not because they were dissatisfied with their home or regarded it as being unsafe. They no longer took their homes for granted.

3.6. Independent but Unprotected

One participant considered a range of alternative places to which he could move, but he had not decided about what he wanted to do. His current home was important to him. This made it difficult for him to move. He also emphasised the following factors: his independence, the substantial effort that he had invested in maintaining his home, the fact that it had a terrace, and his emotional attachment to his home.

H: There was an advertisement where they wanted new tenants. I thought, 'This would be good for me'. I went up to look at it. It's nice. It is one of those terraced house things. There was assistance twenty-four hours a day. I could get food served.
I: Yes.
H: But then, I sit here at night. I have, after all, spent some time on building this conservatory.
I: It's really nice.
H: I just really love this place here.

3.7. Feeling Insecure about Living Alone

When participant H spoke about his feelings of uncertainty and mentioned that he had been looking for a new home, he added:

H: I was a bit scared then. You know, it is a bit difficult for me to get out of this place. I just had no intention of selling; I thought I would rent. But, if I leave here. I couldn't do it.

The female participant (F) described that she was dependent on her husband, and without him she could not cope with her situation at home. Two cancer diagnoses, dizziness and balance problems resulted in her story about feeling insecure in a scenario living alone.

F: My husband helps with all the practical tasks at home.

3.8. Home-Safety Management Collapse

The informants defined to be in the 'home-safety management collapse' theme expressed challenges regarding their life situation and disease progression. They wanted to move because they felt unsafe at home.

3.9. Spending Parts of the Day Alone in the Home

Only two of the eight participants reported that they felt unsafe at home. Both spent considerable parts of their day alone. In both the participants, cancer had resulted in difficulties with mobility and pain. One participant was a woman who was living in a terraced house with her partner. Her partner worked full time and was away during the day. The other participant was a man who lived alone in an apartment on the first floor of a single-family dwelling. His adult son and his partner lived on the ground floor.

D: My husband is at work the whole day.

3.10. High Symptom Burden

The female participant had breast cancer with pelvic and brain metastasis. She reported a long-term disease trajectory, many hospital stays, and long periods where she had endured great difficulties in receiving the necessary help from health care services, especially when the symptoms of the metastasis of breast cancer had emerged. At the time of the interview, her disease status was stable. She had experienced several fractures and undergone several operations (including surgery to stabilise the joints) as a result of her cancer. She had fallen and was injured several times. She reported pain and several symptoms, which can reasonably be attributed to metastasis to the brain. She reported that she felt very unsafe when she was alone at home.

D: . . . back home, here, afterwards, you know, and being alone, when my husband went to work. At the hospital, they would rather get rid of me. They were looking for a place where I could go to stay, and yeah, get some training or something.

After a long process, she was informed that she could stay in a palliative care unit for a few days. She found this solution to be satisfactory.

The other participant, categorized here, was in great pain. He had comorbidities (cancer and diabetes) and complications due to his diseases:

G: All my toes on one of my feet are amputated.

3.11. Unable to Move Around

The latter mentioned male participant who reported feeling unsafe at home expressed a strong desire to move and permanently live in a nursing home. He lived in the same house in which his son was living. His son was away during the day. The participant spent most of his day passively sitting in a chair. He explained that he wished to move because he felt unsafe when he was alone at home and faced challenges when he performed daily tasks. He referred to a respite stay that he had got access to in a nursing home. There he had felt safe and had received the help that he needed.

G: I am not able to move around. I am stuck here in this chair.

4. Discussion

In this study, we examined how older adults with advanced cancer experience their homes, identified the dimensions of their homes that they consider to be important for their home-safety, and investigated the role that cancer plays in the meanings that they assign to their homes. The overarching theme of home-safety management is outlined with three themes.

Theories on late modern societies regard the home as a place that offers shelter and safety. The role that homes play in fostering a sense of security and mental well-being is particularly important because of constant changes in and the occasional unpredictability of societal conditions [16]. Advanced cancer causes unpredictable changes to an individual's abilities, mental health, and experience of their life situation. Accordingly, the need to identify the factors that determine whether older adults feel safe in their own homes has been previously underscored [40]. From this study, we have learned that older adults enjoy living in their homes, and their homes had positive dimensions that enhanced their daily lives. The significant dimensions of the home that were emphasised by the participants were pleasure from the features of their homes, having opportunities to engage in activities, being independent, taking pride in their homes, being grateful for the opportunity to be outdoors, and having access to a garden. Thus, homes can alleviate the negative consequences of cancer and optimize well-being. In such contexts, it is important to conceptualise the relationship between the disease, the mental health status, and the home as a dynamic whole. Specifically, home-safety can relegate cancer to one's mental status, and cancer in turn can make older adults particularly aware of the various valued aspects of their homes. In this regard, the home may serve as a stimulus and represent something positive.

From an older adult's perspective, feelings of safety are an intermediary dimension and condition. For a positive synergy to exist between an older adult and his or her home, he or she must feel safe. The possibility of leading the life that one wishes to live can help older adults feel safe in their own homes [41]. According to Giddens (1991), a sense of safety is related to unconscious psychological aspects. By the overarching theme of home-safety management with its themes and sub-themes, we articulate the role that serious illnesses such as advanced cancer play in one's sense of safety. A sense of safety, which may otherwise be an unconscious and taken-for-granted feeling state, can emerge as an issue that older adults consciously reflect upon and address. Partners play an essential role in this preparatory process. Sharing their homes with their families or partner helped the participants maintain their home, enjoy it, and feel safe in their homes. In this regard, the partners of those with several health issues and those who required substantial assistance made substantial contributions. Their home-safety was maintained because of the contributions of their partners. Concordantly, Aspell et al. (2019) [3] found that the intensity of home support was a predictor of admission to long-term care among home-dwelling older adults. Another study found that older adults in nursing homes feel safer than their home-dwelling counterparts do; this finding is attributable to the easier access to health care personnel [40]. In our study, some participants who lived alone wanted to continue living in their homes, despite facing many difficulties and having health issues. Despite having an advanced disease and a great need for assistance, some older adults felt safe living alone in their own homes.

Decades of research have shown that caring for seriously ill home-dwelling older adults is a great burden to their families [42]. In our study, the partners of some participants had assumed responsibility for home-safety management. Home-safety management can be experienced in different ways and to different extents and can foster a sense of perceived control in older adults. Other studies have shown that maintaining some level of control over one's life when moving into a nursing home influences one's sense of safety [43]. Some older adults recognised and placed substantial emphasis on their dependence on their partner. However, some older adults did not recognise their need for help and dependence, and their partner's contributions were not explicitly acknowledged. Although the partners were responsible for home-safety management, the participants had not explicitly handed over the responsibility to their partners. This may have affected how both parties experienced this situation and contributed to their burden. In accordance with Wahl and Lang's (2006) description of attachment between a person and his or her home, the present findings delineate specific social and emotional dimensions.

Unsurprisingly, some felt uncertain about continuing to live at home. They did not know how their disease could progress and how their life situations might change in the future. When older adults live alone and become dependent on others, uncertainty regarding their home-safety management levels may arise. However, they may not know when and how dependence will happen and what kind of help they will be offered. Thus, he or she is in a moratorium. To a certain degree, they may be aware of their life situation and may think of possible solutions. Several studies have highlighted the particular challenges that are faced by home-dwelling older adults in rural areas who have to travel long distances to receive health care and social services [19,28].

Feeling safe is a precondition for a sense of meaning, mental well-being, and enjoyment of one's home. By conceptualising the home as a space that fosters meaning, safety, and routinised practice, we acknowledge that perceptions of homes are influenced by innumerable experiences that can change in the future [30,44]. Thus, a home has different meanings to different older cancer patients, and these meanings can change with time. A sense of safety and the possibility of maintaining a routinised practice may diminish, depending on personal and household resources and resources in the surroundings. From a recently published article, the authors emphasize discharge planning for end-stage cancer patients [45]. We assume that the same promoting and barrier factors as ethical considerations, and self-efficacy and experience among nurses are also relevant for other countries such as Japan, where discharge planning was studied. A study from Scandinavia shows that good collaboration across health systems [7] has positive effects on the perceived safety of home-dwelling older adults. In our study, some participants felt unsafe even though they shared their homes with their partner or family. This was attributable to prior experiences of difficulties in getting the necessary help, difficulties coping on a daily basis, mobility issues, a fear of falling, and a general sense of uncertainty. The extent of help those older adults require plays a significant role in their sense of safety; severe health issues can reduce their sense of control and, consequently, perceived safety [40]. Thus, receiving proper treatment and care does not guarantee a sense of safety [46].

By examining whether older adults perceive their homes to be spaces within which they feel safe or insecure and unsafe, health care and social services can ascertain the perceived home-safety management levels of older adults. When home-safety management is emphasised, health personnel and social workers should further assess the options that are available to older adults, particularly those with uncertain and collapsed home-safety managements.

The strength of this study is the data collected from a group of home-dwelling older adults with advanced cancer living in different areas in the country (rural and sub-urban municipalities). We did not aim to arrive at generalisable findings. Nevertheless, we acknowledge that using a larger sample may have yielded different results. The sample was sufficiently heterogeneous to facilitate the identification of the significant characteristics of home-safety management. Both male and female older adults with different marital status participated in this study. The participants had extensive and complex health problems. However, we are aware of the difficulties in defining patients to various stages of advanced cancer, as the palliative phase might also include the terminal phase [47]. Based on ethical considerations, we wanted to exclude those most vulnerable cancer patients, defined by us to be in the terminal phase. Through the thematic analysis, the authors engaged in a valuable dialogue, seeking interpretations to understand the data. A limitation in this study is the sample, where patient groups, such as those from ethnic minorities, were not included. The participants were not asked to provide feedback on the results. However, transparent description of the reflexive analytical process should enhance the study's trustworthiness [48]. No software was used for the thematic analysis, and NVivo or other software could have organised the data in a different way than what we did manually.

This study might serve in revealing the generation of hypotheses for further studies. We suggest that studies with large samples should be conducted and studies including urban-dwelling participants.

5. Conclusions

Home-safety management assessment could be an approach to obtain an overview of how home-dwelling older adults with advanced cancer describe their homes, life situation and how the disease impacts their meaning of their home. It is important to adopt a holistic approach to care and pay attention to individual differences in the feelings of being unsafe, which can arise from various situations. We have elaborated on a description of home-safety management and outlined three themes: good home-safety management, uncertain home-safety management, and home-safety management collapse. Modifying the home environment to foster a sense of home-safety may give older adults with advanced cancer the opportunity to experience mental well-being and enjoy living in their homes. This may alleviate the burden of living with cancer.

Author Contributions: Both authors have contributed equally to the project's development, writing the protocol, up-dating the literature review, writing the manuscript, and confirming the manuscript's text. All authors have read and agreed to the published version of the manuscript.

Funding: This study was funded by the Norwegian Cancer Society (grant number 59083001).

Institutional Review Board Statement: The Norwegian Regional Committees for Medical and Health Research Ethics (REK) (REK: #1524) approved this study. https://www.forskningsetikk.no/en/about-us/our-committees-and-commission/rek/ (accessed on 31 December 2012 for the whole project; survey first—documented 2017 and 2020; then interviews—completed 12 December 2017, analyzed 2019–2021. Data is anonymized, i.e., the ID-key is deleted. The anonymized data is available at the SIKT from March 2023).

Informed Consent Statement: Informed consent was obtained from all of the subjects involved in the study.

Data Availability Statement: The data will be stored at the SIKT, previously the Norwegian Social Science Data Services (NSD), after completing the study. https://sikt.no/about-sikt (accessed on 24 October 2022).

Conflicts of Interest: The authors confirm that they have no individual, company, or organization-based interests which involve financial or personal gain.

References

1. WHO. Definition on Mental Health. Available online: https://www.who.int/westernpacific/health-topics/mental-health#tab=tab_1 (accessed on 12 October 2022).
2. Heikkinen, R.-L.; Kauppinen, M. Mental well-being: A 16-year follow-up among older residents in Jyväskylä. *Arch. Gerontol. Geriatr.* **2011**, *52*, 33–39. [CrossRef]
3. Aspell, N.; O'Sullivan, M.; O'Shea, E.; Irving, K.; Duffy, C.; Gorman, R.; Warters, A. Predicting admission to long-term care and mortality among community-based, dependent older people in Ireland. *Int. J. Geriatr. Psychiatry* **2019**, *34*, 999–1007. [CrossRef]
4. Gitlin, L.N. Conducting research on home environments: Lessons learned and new directions. *Gerontologist* **2003**, *43*, 628–637. [CrossRef]
5. Peckham, A.; Rudoler, D.; Li, J.M.; D'souza, S. Community-based reform efforts: The case of the aging at home strategy. *Healthc. Policy* **2018**, *14*, 30. [CrossRef]
6. Wahl, H.-W.; Weisman, G.D. Environmental gerontology at the beginning of the new millennium: Reflections on its historical, empirical, and theoretical development. *Gerontologist* **2003**, *43*, 616–627. [CrossRef] [PubMed]
7. Danielsen, B.V.; Sand, A.M.; Rosland, J.H.; Førland, O. Experiences and challenges of home care nurses and general practitioners in home-based palliative care—A qualitative study. *BMC Palliat. Care* **2018**, *17*, 1–13. [CrossRef] [PubMed]
8. Fjose, M.; Eilertsen, G.; Kirkevold, M.; Grov, E.K. A Valuable but Demanding Time Family Life during Advanced Cancer in an Elderly Family Member. *ANS Adv. Nurs. Sci.* **2016**, *39*, 358–373. [CrossRef]
9. Fjose, M.E.; Kirkevold, G.; Grov, K.E.M. Caregiver reactions and social provisions among family members caring for home-dwelling patients with cancer in the palliative phase: A cross-sectional study. *Clin. Nurs. Stud.* **2019**, *7*, v7n4p1. [CrossRef]
10. Gandarillas, M.Á.; Goswami, N. Merging current health care trends: Innovative perspective in aging care. *Clin. Interv. Aging* **2018**, *13*, 2083. [CrossRef]
11. Schofield, V.; Davey, J.; Keeling, S.; Parsons, M. Ageing in place. In *Implications of Population Ageing: Opportunities and Risks*; Boston, J., Davey, J.A., Eds.; Victoria University of Wellington: Wellington, New Zealand, 2006; pp. 275–306.
12. Roy, N.; Dubé, R.; Després, C.; Freitas, A.; Légaré, F. Choosing between staying at home or moving: A systematic review of factors influencing housing decisions among frail older adults. *PLoS ONE* **2018**, *13*, e0189266. [CrossRef]
13. Barry, A.; Heale, R.; Pilon, R.; Lavoie, A.M. The meaning of home for ageing women living alone: An evolutionary concept analysis. *Health Soc. Care Community* **2018**, *26*, e337–e344. [CrossRef] [PubMed]
14. Massey, D. Space-time, 'science' and the relationship between physical geography and human geography. *Trans. Inst. Br. Geogr.* **1999**, *24*, 261–276. [CrossRef]
15. Wahl, H.-W.; Lang, F.R. Psychological aging: A contextual view. In *Handbook of Models for Human Aging*; Elsevier: Amsterdam, The Netherlands, 2006; pp. 881–895.
16. Giddens, A. *Modernity and Self-Identity, Cambridge*; Polity: Cambridge, UK, 1991; p. 109.
17. Neumann, M.; Wirtz, M.; Ernstmann, N.; Ommen, O.; Längler, A.; Edelhäuser, F.; Scheffer, C.; Tauschel, D.; Pfaff, H. Identifying and predicting subgroups of information needs among cancer patients: An initial study using latent class analysis. *Support. Care Cancer* **2011**, *19*, 1197–1209. [CrossRef] [PubMed]
18. Vallet-Regí, M.; Manzano, M.; Rodriguez-Mañas, L.; Checa López, M.; Aapro, M.; Balducci, L.; Spanish Collaborative Research Network on Aging and Frailty (RETICEF); Barbacid, M.; Guise, T.A.; Balducci, L.; et al. Management of cancer in the older age person: An approach to complex medical decisions. *Oncologist* **2017**, *22*, 335–342. [CrossRef]

19. Fjose, M.; Eilertsen, G.; Kirkevold, M.; Grov, E.K. "Non-palliative care"—A qualitative study of older cancer patients' and their family members' experiences with the health care system. *BMC Health Serv. Res.* **2018**, *18*, 745. [CrossRef]
20. Fitch, M.I.; Coronado, A.C.; Schippke, J.C.; Chadder, J.; Green, E. Exploring the perspectives of patients about their care experience: Identifying what patients perceive are important qualities in cancer care. *Support. Care Cancer* **2020**, *28*, 2299–2309. [CrossRef] [PubMed]
21. Mohile, S.; Dale, W.; Hurria, A. Geriatric oncology research to improve clinical care. *Nat. Rev. Clin. Oncol.* **2012**, *9*, 571–578. [CrossRef]
22. Puts, M.T.; Tapscott, B.; Fitch, M.; Howell, D.; Monette, J.; Wan-Chow-Wah, D.; Krzyzanowska, M.; Leighl, N.B.; Springall, E.; Alibhai, S.M. A systematic review of factors influencing older adults' decision to accept or decline cancer treatment. *Cancer Treat. Rev.* **2015**, *41*, 197–215. [CrossRef]
23. Aoun, S.; Deas, K.; Skett, K. Older people living alone at home with terminal cancer. *Eur. J. Cancer Care* **2016**, *25*, 356–364. [CrossRef]
24. Hanratty, B.; Addington-Hall, J.; Arthur, A.; Cooper, L.; Grande, G.; Payne, S.; Seymour, J. What is different about living alone with cancer in older age? A qualitative study of experiences and preferences for care. *BMC Fam. Pract.* **2013**, *14*, 22. [CrossRef]
25. Wiik, G.B.; Devik, S.; Hellzen, O. Don't become a burden and don't complain: A case study of older persons suffering from incurable cancer and living alone in rural areas. *Nurs. Rep.* **2011**, *1*, 7–14. [CrossRef]
26. Devik, S.A.; Hellzen, O.; Enmarker, I. "Picking up the pieces"—Meanings of receiving home nursing care when being old and living with advanced cancer in a rural area. *Int. J. Qual. Stud. Health Well-Being* **2015**, *10*, 28382. [CrossRef] [PubMed]
27. Keating, N.; Phillips, J. A critical human ecology perspective on rural ageing. In *Rural Ageing: A Good Place Grow Old*; The Policy Press: Bristol, UK, 2008; pp. 1–10.
28. Loughery, J.; Woodgate, R. Supportive care needs of rural individuals living with cancer: A literature review. *Can. Oncol. Nurs. J. Rev. Can. Soins Infirm. Oncol.* **2015**, *25*, 157–166. [CrossRef] [PubMed]
29. Rachakonda, K.; George, M.; Shafiei, M.; Oldmeadow, C. Unmet supportive Cancer care needs: An exploratory quantitative study in rural Australia. *World J. Oncol.* **2015**, *6*, 387. [CrossRef]
30. Gatrell, A. Mobilities and ageing "We're quite outgoing people". In *Geographical Gerontology: Perspectives, Concepts, Approaches*, 1st ed.; Skinner, M.W., Andrews, G.J., Cutchin, M.P., Eds.; Routlegde: London, UK, 2017; p. 350.
31. Mercadante, S.; Aielli, F.; Masedu, F.; Valenti, M.; Ficorella, C.; Porzio, G. Pain characteristics and analgesic treatment in an aged adult population: A 4-week retrospective analysis of advanced cancer patients followed at home. *Drugs Aging* **2015**, *32*, 315–320. [CrossRef]
32. De Boer, D.; Hofstede, J.M.; De Veer, A.J.; Raijmakers, N.J.; Francke, A.L. Relatives' perceived quality of palliative care: Comparisons between care settings in which patients die. *BMC Palliat. Care* **2017**, *16*, 41. [CrossRef]
33. Glenister, D. Creative spaces in palliative care facilities: Tradition, culture, and experience. *Am. J. Hosp. Palliat. Med.* **2012**, *29*, 89–92. [CrossRef]
34. Lang, A.; Toon, L.; Cohen, S.R.; Stajduhar, K.; Griffin, M.; Fleiszer, A.R.; Easty, T.; Williams, A. Client, caregiver, and provider perspectives of safety in palliative home care: A mixed method design. *Saf. Health* **2015**, *1*, 3. [CrossRef]
35. Milberg, A.; Wåhlberg, R.; Jakobsson, M.; Olsson, E.C.; Olsson, M.; Friedrichsen, M. What is a 'secure base' when death is approaching? A study applying attachment theory to adult patients' and family members' experiences of palliative home care. *Psycho-Oncol.* **2012**, *21*, 886–895. [CrossRef] [PubMed]
36. Guldhav, K.V.; Jepsen, R.; Ytrehus, S.; Grov, E.K. Access to information and counselling—Older cancer patients' self-report: A cross-sectional survey. *BMC Nurs.* **2017**, *16*, 18. [CrossRef]
37. Kearns, R.A.; Joseph, A.E. Space in its place: Developing the link in medical geography. *Soc. Sci. Med.* **1993**, *37*, 711–717. [CrossRef]
38. Mason, J. *Qualitative Researching*; Sage: Thousand Oaks, CA, USA, 2017.
39. Braun, V.; Clarke, V. Using thematic analysis in psychology. *Qual. Res. Psychol.* **2006**, *3*, 77–101. [CrossRef]
40. Boström, M.; Bravell, M.E.; Lundgren, D.; Björklund, A. Promoting sense of security in old-age care. *Sci. Rep.* **2013**, *5*, 33178. [CrossRef]
41. Fonad, E.; Wahlin, T.-B.R.; Heikkila, K.; Emami, A. Moving to and living in a retirement home: Focusing on elderly people's sense of safety and security. *J. Hous. Elder.* **2006**, *20*, 45–60. [CrossRef]
42. Golics, C.J.; Basra, M.K.A.; Salek, M.S.; Finlay, A.Y. The impact of patients' chronic disease on family quality of life: An experience from 26 specialties. *Int. J. Gen. Med.* **2013**, *6*, 787. [CrossRef] [PubMed]
43. Stevens, A.K.; Raphael, H.; Green, S.M. A qualitative study of older people with minimal care needs experiences of their admission to a nursing home with Registered Nurse care. *Qual. Ageing Older Adults* **2015**, *16*, 94–105. [CrossRef]
44. Somerville, P. The social construction of home. *J. Archit. Plan. Res.* **1997**, *14*, 226–245.
45. Aoyanagi, M.; Shindo, Y.; Takahashi, K. General Ward Nurses' Self-Efficacy, Ethical Behavior, and Practice of Discharge Planning for End-Stage Cancer Patients: Path Analysis. *Healthcare* **2022**, *10*, 1161. [CrossRef]
46. Schwappach, D.L.; Wernli, M. Am I (un) safe here? Chemotherapy patients' perspectives towards engaging in their safety. *Qual. Saf. Health Care* **2010**, *19*, e9. [CrossRef]
47. Grov, E.K. The Cancer trajectory—A model of phases. *Vård Nord. Nord. J. Nurs. Res.* **2014**, *34*, 46–47. [CrossRef]
48. Lincoln, Y.S.; Guba, E.G. *Naturalistic Inquiry*; Sage Publication: Thousand Oaks, CA, USA, 1985.

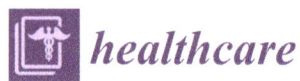

Article

The Psychological Distress and Quality of Life of Breast Cancer Survivors in Sydney, Australia

Laura-Anne Aitken and Syeda Zakia Hossan *

Faculty of Medicine and Health, The University of Sydney, Camperdown, NSW 2006, Australia
* Correspondence: zakia.hossain@sydney.edu.au; Tel.: +61-2-935-19340

Abstract: In Australia, breast cancer is one of the most common cancers affecting women. Between 1987–1991 and 2012–2016, the five-year survival rate improved from 75% to 91%. The increased chance of survival due to early detection and treatment interventions has resulted in more women living with the diagnosis. This qualitative study was designed to analyse the journey of breast cancer survivors, their experience of psychological distress and changes in quality of life (QOL) due to the increased prevalence amongst Australian women. In-depth interviews were conducted; they lasted over 45 min and comprised 15 participants. The main topics discussed were knowledge of breast cancer prior to diagnosis, psychological distress, QOL and experience of use of healthcare services. The results showed that the process of diagnosis, undergoing treatment and isolation post-treatment resulted in high amounts of psychological distress. A reduction in QOL was also experienced due to treatment and medication side effects, fatigue, cognitive changes, and body-image perception. These findings can assist researchers in providing evidence-based frameworks for policy changes and for further investigation into effective healthcare interventions.

Keywords: breast cancer; psychological distress; quality of life; women's health; qualitative study

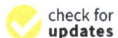

Citation: Aitken, L.-A.; Hossain, S.Z. The Psychological Distress and Quality of Life of Breast Cancer Survivors in Sydney, Australia. *Healthcare* **2022**, *10*, 2017. https://doi.org/10.3390/healthcare10102017

Academic Editor: Margaret Fitch

Received: 22 September 2022
Accepted: 11 October 2022
Published: 12 October 2022

Publisher's Note: MDPI stays neutral with regard to jurisdictional claims in published maps and institutional affiliations.

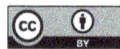

Copyright: © 2022 by the authors. Licensee MDPI, Basel, Switzerland. This article is an open access article distributed under the terms and conditions of the Creative Commons Attribution (CC BY) license (https://creativecommons.org/licenses/by/4.0/).

1. Introduction

Breast cancer is one of the most common causes of cancer-related deaths in women globally. It occurs when abnormal cells in the breast grow uncontrollably. It is more common among women; however, a small proportion of men also are affected by breast cancer [1]. After diagnosis, some common treatments that Breast Cancer Survivors (BCS) receive are a lumpectomy, mastectomy, chemotherapy or hormone therapy [2]. Due to the raised awareness and focus on early detection programs, survival is becoming increasingly likely for breast cancer patients [3]. Within Australia, breast cancer in 2016 was the most common cancer affecting women, with 330 new cases per 100,000 people [4]. Between 1987–1991 and 2012–2016, the five-year survival rate improved from 75% to 91%, increasing the number of survivors in the community [4]. This is due to increased awareness campaigns and breast screening availability provided by companies, including BreastScreen Australia [5]. BreastScreen Australia is the state and territory initiative of the Australian government to increase early detection and thus decrease illness and death. It allows women over 40 to have a free mammogram every two years [6].

For BCS, common issues range from treatment side effects [5], financial hardships [7] and comorbidities [8] to social isolation [9]. Many studies have assessed the health related QOL of BCS [5,10–12]; however, there is limited research that focuses on Australian women who have survived cancer and continue to experience its detrimental effects. QOL and psychological distress are essential patient-centred outcomes, assisting with assessing cancer care delivery. BCS is a medical and social label for all who live with cancer diagnosis until death, irrespective of the cause [13]. These BCS undergo considerable stress and trauma throughout diagnosis, treatment and post-treatment, which continues even after survival, subsequently impacting their QOL. The main factors identified in the literature as the significant causes of stress and trauma include psychological distress, financial stress and social isolation.

Studies have indicated that BCS experience mental health issues as soon as they are diagnosed with cancer, during treatment and survivorship. Two main concerns within psychological distress have been identified for BCS: mental health issues and distress surrounding cognitive function. One-fourth of breast cancer patients will develop anxiety and depression at some point in the breast cancer journey [14]. Those aged younger than 50 years are especially likely to report psychological distress [15,16] compared to the older cohort aged > 50 years. However, it is also said that 12 months post-diagnosis, most BCS have returned to pre-diagnosis levels of distress [17]. This discrepancy between studies highlights the importance of a study to outline mental health issues throughout the journey, rather than just certain checkpoints.

QOL is an individual's perception of their position in life, in the context of the culture and value system they live within along with their goals, expectations, standards and concerns [18]. It is clear from the review of the literature that various stressors have resulted in a reduction in QOL for BCS. Previous research on QOL has focused on understanding the QOL in the early phases of breast cancer and groups of older BCS [10]. Most of these studies, however, focused on survivors 10 years post-diagnosis. The conclusions drawn were similar, with the participants reporting low QOL with additional sexuality, pain and psychological distress issues. This was illustrated in a quantitative study with BCS between the ages of 40 and 49, which found that the presence of breast-related symptoms at the time of survey completion had a profound impact on QOL [5].

Within the literature, there is insufficient focus on the qualitative experience of Australian BCS from diagnosis to survivorship. Most of the literature available is based on quantitative studies, with limited research being available on the experiences of BCS. This research is an attempt to fill this gap. There has also been a focus on mental health and cognitive disorders such as struggles with depression and increased anxiety; However, there is a need for a greater understanding of the progression of these issues in Australian BCS throughout their entire BC journey.

This research aims to understand the journey undergone by BCS diagnosed with breast cancer from diagnosis to survivorship. Furthermore, it explores the challenges experienced by the BCS due to physical changes, financial hardship, emotional distress and social isolation The Australian healthcare system is unique due to the country's cultural diversity and different demographics. Understanding the experience of specifically Australian women with breast cancer is essential, as it will allow healthcare providers to understand the experiences of BCS in greater depth within the cultural context. This, in turn, may help facilitate greater sensitivity when treating their patients and assist in developing strategies and policies for BCS.

This cross-sectional exploratory research is based on a qualitative research method. It aims to understand the journey undergone by women, diagnosed with breast cancer, from diagnosis to survivorship. Further, it explores the challenges experienced by the BCS due to physical change, financial hardship, emotional distress and social isolation.

2. Materials and Methods

Eligible participants were BCS; they were aged 35 years and above, living in Sydney and had been diagnosed for at least a year. A total of 15 women with breast cancer were recruited for the study. Participants were excluded if they had been diagnosed less than one year ago to ensure all participants had completed their treatment. Participants that were diagnosed greater than 11 years prior were also excluded as they may not clearly recollect their early experience of diagnosis. Multiple strategies were used to recruit participants including snowball and convenience sampling, social media and community organisation advertising. For example, through the assistance of the organisation Pink Hope, a preventative health charity, we acquired participants using flyers. Advertising on social media gained the most traction, with participants sharing and passing on information to other survivors. Before recruitment commenced, ethics approval was obtained from the University of Sydney Human Research Ethics Committee (25 August 2021). The participants were also presented with the "Participant Information Statement" to ensure the study had informed consent and that participation was entirely voluntary and anonymous. The data were also saved in OneDrive and password-protected, and only researchers had access. These in-depth interviews were conducted over 45 min with 15 BCS. The first author participated in two days of training prior to the interviews commencing.

This specific qualitative method was chosen to ensure that the full experience of BCS was explored effectively. In particular, QOL was measured subjectively rather than using established measurement tools. Quantitative measurement of QOL qualifies experience's on a scale rather than exploring participants' experiences which was important for this study. In the in-depth interviews, the interviewer led the BCS through a series of open-ended questions to establish the experience of breast cancer diagnosis, treatment and living with the diagnosis (Appendix A). The interviews were conducted over 3 weeks in August and September 2021 and were recorded via Zoom. These in-depth interviews allow the participant to determine the direction of the interview and are, therefore, an effective method for an exploratory study [19].

A thematic analysis was conducted by researchers on the interviews [20]. Firstly, each interview was transcribed. An excel document was then prepared with each of the interview questions as titles. The responses from every participant relating to that question were then compiled for easy comparison. The first author then went through each response and highlighted common words and phrases used by the participants. These words and phrases were then grouped together to form the codes for each question. These codes were used to identify the common themes and to identify similarities between the BCS journeys.

3. Results

The main themes identified within this study were emotional and psychological distress throughout the journey of BCS, a reduction in QOL seen through social changes and physical symptoms and access to health services.

3.1. Background Information

3.1.1. Sociodemographic Background

The sociodemographic background of the study participants is presented in Table 1. The average age of the study participants is 45 years, the youngest being aged 35 years. Participants had received their diagnosis between 1 and 11 years prior to the study. On average, 66% of participants were employed with education levels ranging from year 12 graduation to tertiary studies. The majority (80%) of participants were married and had between 1 and 4 children (See Table 1).

3.1.2. Previous Knowledge of Breast Cancer

Participants were asked to recount the knowledge they had of symptoms, diagnosis and treatment of breast cancer prior to their diagnosis. Three participants had a family history of breast cancer and were more likely to be informed about breast cancer. Symptoms identified by the participants were lumps, swelling, sensitivity and pain in the breast. Around 66.7% of participants had heard of a mammogram before, and 40% knew of breast self-examination (BSE). The most common treatment identified was chemotherapy, with 73.3% reporting prior knowledge (see Table 2). Some of the comments by the study participant's symptoms, diagnosis and treatment of breast cancer are presented in Table 2.

Table 1. Sociodemographic Background.

Variables	Subgroups	% (n)
Age (average = 45)	35–39	26.6 (4)
	40–45	20(3)
	46–49	6.6 (1)
	50–55	13.3 (2)
	56–60	13.3 (2)
Employment Status	Fulltime	20 (3)
	Part-time/casual	46 (7)
	Unemployed	33.3 (5)
Level of Education	High School	26.6 (4)
	Tertiary studies	
	- Diploma	26.6 (4)
	- Graduate Certificate	6.67 (1)
	- Undergraduate	13.3 (2)
	- Postgraduate	26.6 (4)
Religion	Christian	66.67 (10)
	No Religion	26.6 (4)
	Muslim	6.67 (1)
Marital Status	Married	80 (12)
	Divorced	6.66 (1)
	Single	6.67 (1)
	De-facto	6.67 (1)
Family Income	20,000–50,000	13.3 (2)s
	50,000–100,000	26.6 (4)
	100,000–150,000	6.67 (1)
	150,000–200,000	26.6 (4)
	200,000+	20 (3)
Children	0	6.67 (1)
	1–2	53.3 (8)
	3–4	33.3 (5)
Country of Birth	Australian	80 (12)
	Argentina	6.67 (1)
	India	6.67 (1)
	Bangladesh	6.67 (1)

Table 2. Breast cancer previous knowledge.

Q: What did You Know about the Symptoms of Breast Cancer?		Q: What did You Know about How to Diagnose Breast Cancer?		Q: Did You Know How Breast Cancer was Treated?	
Example Responses		Example Responses		Example Responses	
"If you feel a lump or anything abnormal sort of on your chest or under your armpit, sort of self-examining that way" (P 005)		"My mother had had breast cancer ... GP was very conservative ... I would walk in and have a mammogram and an ultrasound every year since I was 40" (P015)		"Well, I knew obviously, chemotherapy was gonna be usually ... Other than surgery, chemotherapy is usually the first medical treatment after surgery, and then I knew, obviously, radiation as well. I didn't know all the in-depth parts of having to get set up for all those treatments, but I knew about those treatments" (P011)	
As I always had thought, it would be like a lump. I was always had the breast cancer described as being a lump, like a pea or like a stone" (P007)		"I hadn't done any mammograms or ultrasounds before. And to be honest, I'd never checked myself really, ever. I think I maybe did a couple of times, but it wasn't something every month like you're supposed to. So yeah, I didn't do that" (P010)		"Well, I thought it was literally just either surgery or chemo like that two options, that's really it. But didn't realise how much options within each of those there were as well, yeah" (P003)	
		Common Phrases % (n)			
Lump	66.67 (10)	Self-Check	40 (6)	Surgery	33.3 (5)
Changes	13.3 (2)	Dr. Check	20 (3)	Mastectomy	20 (2)
None	20 (3)	Mammogram	66.67 (10)	Chemotherapy	73.3 (11)
		Ultrasound	20 (3)	Radiation	46.67 (7)
		Biopsy	6.67 (1)	None	20 (3)
		None	13.3 (2)		

3.1.3. Diagnosis of Breast Cancer

Participants were asked, "How did you find out you had breast cancer?" The three main methods of diagnosis were finding a breast lump through self-examination, noticing changes in their breasts and through ultrasounds and mammograms. Approximately 40% mentioned that, initially, they dismissed the symptoms as being hormonal or something less serious (See Table 3).

3.1.4. Treatment of Breast Cancer

Of these 15 participants, the most common sources of treatment reported were chemotherapy, radiation and surgery. Out of the total participants, 86.6% had chemotherapy and 53% had radiation, and all the participants underwent surgery (the majority received a mastectomy 66.6%). Side effects from these treatments and the preventative medications were also highly reported to impact QOF (See Table 4).

Table 3. Experience of Breast Cancer. How did you find out you had breast cancer?

Keywords	% (n)	Responses
Self-check to find lump	46.67 (7)	"I actually felt and saw the lump. I was just doing a little, not spring clean, but just moving little things around and yes, found a lump form, tried to massage it, didn't go away and sort of went to my GP to check it out" (P005)
Changes in breast	33.3 (5)	"I just woke up one morning and had a swollen breast, one swollen breast that was a little bit tender. [chuckle] And it was a little strange, it was different for me, but it was also something that I was going to quickly dismiss and pretty much did really, 'cause it went away within two days" (P003)
Pain	20 (3)	"I was in the shower one morning and I kind of leant over to wash myself and I felt a pain kinda of in the side of my breast on the left, then I felt there and there was a distinct lump" (P009)
Dismissed symptoms (hormonal)	40 (6)	"Anyway, I had a ... Early in the year, I did go and see my GP to say, 'Something really doesn't sort of feel quite right', but I was completely just putting it down to hormonal, to relative to hormonal changes" (P007)
Fast diagnosis and movement to treatment	33.3 (5)	"Went to the doctor straight away. So I think within two days, I had an appointment with the doctor. From there, I went and had a mammogram and an ultrasound. He got me into the specialist very, very quickly, I had a biopsy at the specialist, I saw the specialist, I had breast cancer. So within ... I think within probably two weeks" (P009)
Mammogram + ultrasound	60 (9)	
Misdiagnosed/long diagnosis process	20 (3)	"Doctor on board Queen Victoria said, 'I think you're crazy, you don't need to go back. I thought you've already been cleared, you don't need a biopsy' ... took them two years for them to diagnose me on board Queen Victoria, and by then I'd seen five of their doctors and I had reported with each of the doctors saying, 'Oh, this couldn't possibly be any problem, and it couldn't possibly need a biopsy. She's just too young.'" (P006)

Table 4. Treatments % (n).

Mastectomy	80 (12)
Chemotherapy	93.3 (14)
Radiation	53.3 (8)
Reconstruction	26.67 (4)
Lumpectomy	13.3 (2)
Oncoplastic Resection	6.67 (1)
Hysterectomy	20 (3)

3.2. Psychological and Emotional Distress

The study participants were asked to share any experience they had of psychological or emotional distress. Open-ended questions were used to assist participants in outlining their experience during diagnosis, treatment and post-treatment. Responses were categorised under the broad themes and presented below:

3.2.1. Experience of Receiving Diagnosis and Treatment of Breast Cancer

Most participants (46%) went into a state of shock when they received their diagnosis, with three of the fifteen participants reporting a memory loss or blurred memories of the moment and four others reporting a trauma response (hot flushes, anxiety). Participant 010 described the experience as:

"My whole world just collapsed. And I think I just sat in his room for like 20 min wailing, feeling like I was gonna be sick."

Three of the fifteen participants reported crying, while four mentioned moving into "survival mode" to attack the problem pragmatically. Participant 008 stated that:

"First question was, out of my mouth was what are we doing about it? Tell me what to do next ... I was very practical, very pragmatic."

3.2.2. Treatment: Chemotherapy, Surgery and Radiation

Of the 15 BCS interviewed, 13 went through at least one round of chemotherapy, either pre- or post-surgery. About 40% of participants reported a feeling of losing their identity, and 33% reported feeling helpless. For example, participant 015 stated that:

> "Chemo is terrible 'cause you lose not just your hair, you lose your eyelashes and your eyebrows, you lose absolutely everything . . . you just go grey, and again, it is the treatment that makes you sick . . . I found it overwhelming at times, I was quite emotional."

3.2.3. Post-Treatment

After treatment had been completed, several BCS reported a lack of direction and support, which caused psychological distress. Due to the continuing side effects of medications, menopause and the abrupt nature of ending treatment, 40% of BCS report of feeling abandoned and isolated.

> "I have had such a long time of treatment and now, I feel like I am going into this open water of not as much intensity." (P010)

Participant 011 also described the inability to deal with long-term medication side effects that caused considerable distress in many BCS.

> "There is always an end in sight . . . you have the surgery, and then you want clear margins, and you get your diagnosis . . . You know how many treatments of chemotherapy you are having over a period of time, You know how many treatments of radiation you are having over a period of time. So, once you get through all of that they put you on this medication, which the side effects don't end . . . There is no end in sight." (P011)

3.2.4. Anxious for Recurrence

A common phrase repeated amongst participants was "scanxiety" (3 participants), which describes the feeling of panic and stress before a check-up and scan. BCS also report a hyper awareness of aches and pains and how they jump to the conclusion of cancer quickly (46%). Four BCS described this anxiety as always being in the back of their minds and as constant stress. Participant 008 especially struggled with this stress and described her experience:

> "Biggest thing that I battle with all the time, it's always there. It may not rear its ugly head every day, but it is always at the back of your mind, always." (P008)

3.3. Quality of Life

Open-ended questions were asked about the impact of breast cancer on the QOL of the study participants. These questions focused on daily activities, sleep, fatigue, cognition, physical body image and sexuality. The three main themes that contributed to changes in QOL were physical symptoms, support network issues and finally accessibility to services.

3.3.1. Physical Symptoms

Several common symptoms impacted the QOL of BCS. These included the inability to sleep, increased fatigue, chemo fog, vaginal dryness and changes in body image. Almost all BCS reported having issues with the perception of their bodies. The majority reported embarrassment of their bodies, particularly how they look in front of others, feeling unattractive to partners and a reduction in self-esteem. Five of the study participants highlighted concerns with the reconstructions, while three BCS outlined how not having nipples contributed to this issue. Participant 006 linked her issues with body image to her relationship with her husband and her sexuality.

> "Now it is just very obvious I don't have nipples, but they are just it looks like I've been massacred. And my husband is a bit sad about it all [chuckle].

Unfortunately, men are very . . . They're quite visual creatures, unfortunately, in my experience, from what I've seen, but he's very understanding, and I think it's more the problem of the menopause, which is why sex life is dwindling." (P006)

Some BCS did report that cutting off their own hair before it fell out was a way to regain some control.

"I did make a pre-emptive strike to cut off my hair, but not straight away, 'cause I used to have really long, curly hair, and I thought, Well, that's something . . . Like I think a lot of women, something you can control." (P007)

Difficulties sleeping were reported by 66% of the BCS, while the other four participants had no issues with sleeping. Four BCS mentioned that hot flushes and side effects from menopause are the reason for this poor sleep, whereas two others associated poor sleep with an overactive mind. Three BCS use sleeping tablets and melatonin to get to sleep.

"So not very good sleep to begin with and the chemo, I couldn't sleep, I couldn't . . . I just felt sick the whole time. Trying to sleep when you're feeling nausea, wasn't fun, so it was very difficult trying to sleep and then getting up and smells really affected me." (P014)

Fatigue not only impacts BCS during chemotherapy but lasts for years post-treatment. Three women reported that they feel like they have less energy, and two others say they have issues with maintaining work-hour requirements. On average, fatigue was worse during treatment, and now most BCS have reported improvements. Participant 009 was one of many BCS who experienced issues returning to work due to fatigue.

"I would say for the first three years the fatigue is really, really tangible, very hard to, I guess, to sustain things for a long period of time . . . I found working, going back to work, even though it was a couple of days a week at first, were exhausting. Now, I still, even now, I still don't have the physical, I guess, stamina that I used to have." (P009)

Cognitive changes impact self-confidence and workability. BCS have reported feeling like they can't remember words and suffer from chemo fog and short-term memory loss. Four of these participants are worried about these cognitive changes impacting their working life. This issue was highlighted by participant 002, who stated:

"As well, so I think once I got back into that, I felt like my brain came back online, but before that, It's like I could. Sometimes I couldn't even find the words to say, and I was worried. I'm like how am I gonna go back to work and have these conversations with families? And you know, I sound dumb pretty much." (P002)

Bodily changes due to menopause, medication side effects and changes in self-esteem have been seen to reduce BCS ability to be intimate. For varying reasons, from the experience of dryness and pain to a lower libido, 60% of the participants reported some change in their sex lives. Participant 009 describes her struggle with getting hormone replacement therapy to reduce symptoms and improve her ability to be intimate.

"I had a very healthy sex life with my husband before any of this happened. Now it is non-existent. Not fun, not wanting to. But it is extremely painful. It doesn't . . . I can't obviously, can't take HRT, I have tried. I have begged, I have screened, I have fought with doctors, I've been shut down at every turn." (P009)

Another participant outlined the steps she has taken to improve her sexual functioning.

"Firstly, you don't really feel like it, that's for sure. But then afterwards, I think because of menopause, you've dryness and discomfort, definitely suffering from both of those. But because of my involvement volunteering with The Mater, I was lucky enough in those groups . . . So, she talked us through the option of laser in your cervix to get that sort of moisture back. But I . . . So we need to use lubricant now because it's never really got back to 100% normal." (P008)

3.3.2. Support Systems

Support system changes were identified in the breast cancer survivors' relationships with their children, husbands, friends and family members. These changes not only impacted them emotionally during the time of treatment but have also had lasting effects post-treatment. Most of these BCS (80%) were married and had children, and a majority of them reported that their husbands were extremely supportive.

> "He was very supportive. I was very lucky. I you know on being on breast cancer support group pages that I so many stories of relationships breaking down and you know divorce and all the rest of it. But yeah, no I was very lucky he was 100% in it with me." (P002)

A few BCS did outline issues with children's behaviour or difficulties amongst the extended family unit. Participant 014 in particular noted the difficulties within a family unit.

> "My little girl was quite young at the time, so she didn't really know what was going on, but her behaviour started becoming quite bad during it all ... So it was difficult for the older kinds, but they all worked so they threw themselves into work and study and friends and kind of like, I felt like they ignored me a lot." (P014)

Seven out of the fifteen participants' social networks shifted during their journey. Three BCS highlighted their desire for privacy throughout this time, while three others mentioned that they felt forgotten. Six BCS specifically mentioned that they felt disconnected and distant. Alternatively, 33% of BCS reported not feeling isolated and completely supported by their community, family and friends

For participant 008, it came as a surprise as to who stepped up and who stepped back.

> "I felt like my network went into the washing machine and some people went down the drain, and others who came out lovely and fluffy; they are my posse. I'd trust my life with them. It's quite amazing the people who step away ... But I had a couple of very, very close friends who are not in my inner circle anymore, and just stepped away." (P008)

3.4. Health Services Experience

BCS in both the public and private sectors reported financial distress throughout their journey (see Table 5). Out of the 15 participants, only 5 reported not having financial stress during this time. Of these BCS, all five were part of the private health system. Many did, however, acknowledge the steep prices and shock felt over the cost of their treatment, commenting that they were "lucky" to be able to afford treatment. Of the BCS experiencing financial stress, three were in the public system, and five were private. One woman highlighted the stress of having a lack of income on her family:

Table 5. Financial Stress and Healthcare System.

	Financial Distress n (%)	No Financial Distress (n)
Public System	3 (20%)	0
Private System	5 (33%)	5 (33%)
No comment	2 (13%)	

> "My husband had to take time off because he had to return to his work. The cancer therapy helped us pay half the bill, which they do because of the stress that comes on between a family and then the kids trying to go to school, go to work, and then your husband's gotta look after the little one, cook, clean and wash." (P012)

There were also reports that post-treatments, due to financial constraints, BCS were not able to access services to improve their QOL.

"Everything that's come after it is virtually out of pocket so that I can't afford to seek the therapy that I actually really need on a regular basis." (P007)

During treatment, interactions with the medical staff and ease of using services contributed to the overall QOL of BCS. One woman mentioned that she felt "like everyone was treating me like a queen. It was great. I'm like everyone so nice to me because they know I've got cancer" (P002), whereas another mentioned that during treatment she had a few issues with communication that led to further anxiety.

"Oh, you've got more of a chance of it coming back somewhere else than in the other breast", and I remember thinking, "Did you just hear what you just said?" They just . . . I know it's hard for them and they need to be separate emotionally, but they also need to remember that they're dealing with people and they're dealing with people's lives"

As mentioned previously, there was a drop-off in support after active treatment. Here, BCS reported that they had difficulty getting help for the side effects of medications.

"They don't give you any way to manage those symptoms of what you're gonna go through on the medication. They don't identify things that you can go, "Oh, that's what that is, and this is how I can treat it, how to avoid it." They just kind of ignore the fact that you have side effects from it, or they say, "You know, I've seen people worse off, so you've got it okay." (P011)

4. Discussion

This study revealed that participants frequently reported psychological distress and a reduction in QOL. This aligns with the previous literature, where issues of financial hardships [7], comorbidities [8] and social isolation [9] were reported. The most prevalent issues highlighted by these studies BCS were the harm of the side effects from post-treatment medication, anxiety around cancer recurrence and issues with health service utilisation.

Psychological distress is the emotional suffering associated with stressors and demands that are difficult to cope with daily. The results from this study illustrate that the significant points of psychological distress along the journey of BCS are receiving the diagnosis during treatment and, finally, the process of survivorship. The most commonly endorsed stressors include chemotherapy trauma (46%) and loss of identity (40%). The anxiety of reoccurrence was noted by all survivors, with three of the fifteen participants reporting that it no longer concerns them. The literature has observed that BCS levels of anxiety and depression decrease over time, which contradicts the findings of our study where it has increased [21]. The increase in distress during the transition from active treatment aligns with qualitative and anecdotal studies [22], whereas contradicting quantitative studies report a decrease in distress at this time [23,24]. There were three main events where psychological distress occurred for BCS. These included receiving the diagnosis, completing treatment and post treatment abandonment which have also been observed in other studies [25,26]. When diagnosed, participants went into a state of shock and experienced trauma responses. Four of the fifteen participants did, however, mention that their first instinct was to attack the problem pragmatically. The next source of distress was going through treatment, especially chemotherapy. Side effects such as losing hair and the feeling of helplessness were significant contributors to psychological distress. Finally, post-treatment feelings of abandonment by the healthcare system and the lack of direction also contributed to distress, which is supported by a growing body of evidence [27,28]. Here, it was evident that participants felt abandoned and struggled with not having any support networks to assist with the transition.

Participants' QOL was explored by discussing how certain indicators, identified from the literature review, have impacted participants' QOL. The significant concerns derived from these interviews were physical symptoms of BC, changes in support systems for BCS and poor body-image perception.

Poor body image is associated with mastectomies and breast reconstruction surgery [11]. Although a smaller sample was used, this study supported those findings. Over half of the BCS reported a drop in self-esteem, feeling unattractive to partners and embarrassed by their breasts. There was a consensus amongst two of the BCS claiming to be unsatisfied with their reconstruction, often suggesting that they struggle with having or not having tattooed nipples. Survivors have reported sexual health concerns for up to 10 years post-treatment [29]. In Pumo et al.'s (2012) study, sexual conditions that directly correlated to psychological disorders were prevalent in 36% of their participants [30]. Within this study, sexual issues and complications such as dryness, pain and low libido to side effects of treatments were linked with medications rather than psychological disorders. There were also reports of participants' embarrassment of how they look affecting their desire to be intimate with their partner.

Sleep and fatigue are both factors contributing to the reduction in QOL. Several BCS reported insomnia, trouble staying asleep and extreme fatigue throughout the day. There was a common trend of fatigue and sleep issues being more prevalent during treatment and then improving as time went on, supported in the literature [31]. There was, however, a few BCS that reported persistent trouble sleeping and fatigue even years post-treatment. In Beck et al.'s 2010 study, this trend was also seen where some survivors continued to experience problems with sleep many years later [32]. This constant fatigue has resulted in reducing the workability of survivors and the ability to spend time with families, which has led to a reduction in QOL.

Cognitive changes were linked to memory loss and reduced capacity for work for the majority of the study participants. Similar findings were reported in previous studies, where participants noticed language, memory, spatial ability and motor function changes [33]. However, there was some discrepancy among participants regarding whether the medication, treatment or effects of ageing were causing the changes in cognition. Collins et al. (2009) discussed this phenomenon concerning hormonal therapies such as tamoxifen and anastrozole [34]. It was concluded that hormonal therapies subtly have a negative influence on cognition. This aligned with our findings as the negative side effects of tamoxifen were mentioned by four of the fifteen participants and linked to their cognitive changes and other physical symptoms. There were also conversations linking these cognitive changes to stressors in the workplace, with BCS worrying that it would affect their performance. Similar findings were cited in Nelson and Sul's (2013) study, which noted that the detrimental effects of reduced memory and learning impacted the workplace and function roles [35].

The majority of participants were married and had children. This resulted in extensive conversations about relationship changes and social isolation. Most BCS reported that their husbands were highly supportive and a great help during this time. Only a minority mentioned relationship breakdowns and increased stress due to their partners. Multiple studies have illustrated the positive effect of supportive spousal relationships [36,37], which our study supports. Even with this support, many BCS still feel isolated post-treatment due to a lack of continued understanding of their experience from family and friends [38] and continued side effects of medications. Perz et al. (2013) explored that the heightened fear of rejection experienced by BCS with potential partners causes survivors to isolate themselves even further [39]. The single woman who participated in this study reported that they felt embarrassed by their breast appearance; however, this fear of rejection was not explicitly mentioned. There was also no mention of participants further isolating themselves as they sought out more connections via social networks, support groups and their own families. Those who had better support networks of friends, family and communities mentioned that going through treatment was easier with all the extra help, and thus they felt less isolated. When this community was not present, there were often reports of feeling helpless and overwhelmed by tasks. This is supported in the literature, where those who have strong relationships and communities to assist them felt protected from negative feelings such as depression, anxiety and the stigma of BC [9,36,38].

The experience of using and accessing healthcare services was identified as a significant factor contributing to QOL. Within Australia, Medicare is the publicly funded universal health care insurance scheme that all Australians can access. In addition to this, private health coverage is also available to paying customers to cover the gaps in Medicare. These two services however still do not alleviate the entire financial burden of Breast Cancer treatments and services. Financial distress acted as a significant barrier to healthcare services for BCS [40]. This result was expected because various studies outlined expensive costs and lack of coverage via Medicare and private health [40]. The previous literature also outlined that breast cancer comorbidities would also be a barrier to returning to work [41], which was also seen in this study. One central area discussed was the difficulties affording services post-treatment. Through the public and private health sectors, most women received some financial support.

In some cases, participants had to pick and choose the most needed services at a specific time rather than having access to all services that may improve their QOL. Although the majority did report that financially they were stable, all acknowledge the exorbitant costs of life-saving and life-enhancing treatments during survivorship. Breast reconstruction was a significant source of financial strain. It is not covered under Medicare, and as it is not considered a life-saving surgery, private health services often do not cover it.

Treatment and communication by staff within the healthcare system had a significant impact on survivors' experience and distress. Four of the fifteen BCS reported at least one issue of switching practitioners or feeling like they were not being heard. One of the most considerable contributions to distress during diagnosis was the communication of medical staff about the severity and course of action for treatments. Participants also highlighted how their health was now in their own hands after treatment, and there was no transition phase. Many felt abandoned and isolated by the shift in control as well as being at a loss as to how to manage their symptoms into the future. Most participants continued to take medication after their treatments to prevent cancer recurrence. These medications, however, had harmful side effects that BCS have had to learn how to manage by themselves. This, paired with financial restrictions, has resulted in a reduction in QOL.

However, there are a few limitations of the study. The limitations of this study include social media and readiness bias. The effectiveness of social media recruitment resulted in a biased sample toward BCS who do not use or do not have access to social media. In addition, it also eliminates participants who are not yet ready to share their experiences as they are still dealing with the consequences of their disease.

5. Summary and Conclusions

Fifteen BCS were interviewed to understand their journey from pre-diagnosis to survivorship. The average participants were aged 35–45, had at least one child, were married and were Australian. The most common issues mentioned throughout this study were the lack of interventions for medication side effects, changes in their body image and anxiety around cancer reoccurrence. There were also many accounts of how physical side effects from treatments have impacted their work and social and sexual lives.

These findings are based on a qualitative study, with a small sample of 15 in-depth interviews; therefore, a generalisation of the study cannot be made. Due to the small number of participants and sampling error, there was also a lack of older participants from diverse backgrounds.

This study has provided a preliminary basis for the experience of BCS and can expanded on in a larger study using quantitative methods to assess QOL and psychological distress. These findings have implications for policymakers and for the healthcare industry along with the importance of a survivor's relationship with their healthcare team and their ability to access services, which was especially highlighted. It would be our recommendation to focus future studies on the experience of BCS from ages 35 to 45 including their diagnosis. Future studies should also include BCS of culturally diverse groups and older age cohorts.

From this research, it is also clear that younger women should have access to free and convenient mammograms. Additionally, the experience of sexuality and early menopause is an area that needs to be examined to provide better services and support for survivors. Access to post-care services, links to support groups and information about medication side effects should be prioritised in order to increase survivors' QOL.

Author Contributions: Here are the contributions from authors: Conceptualization, S.Z.H.; methodology S.Z.H. and L.-A.A.; software, L.-A.A.; validation, S.Z.H. and L.-A.A.; formal analysis, L.-A.A. and S.Z.H.; investigation, L.-A.A. and S.Z.H.; resources, S.Z.H. and L.-A.A.; data curation, L.-A.A. and S.Z.H.; writing—original draft preparation, L.-A.A.; writing—review and editing, L.-A.A. and S.Z.H.; supervision, S.Z.H.; project administration, S.Z.H. and L.-A.A. All authors have read and agreed to the published version of the manuscript.

Funding: This research received no external funding.

Institutional Review Board Statement: The study was conducted in accordance with the Human Research Ethics Committee of the University of Sydney (Protocol number 2021/525 and date 18 August 2021.

Informed Consent Statement: Informed consent was obtained from all subjects involved in the study.

Conflicts of Interest: The authors declare no conflict of interest.

Appendix A

	Section 1: Breast Cancer Diagnosis: Treatment and Experience
1.1	Can you tell us how much you knew about breast cancer prior to your diagnosis?
(a)	What did you know about the symptoms of breast cancer?
(b)	What did you know about how to diagnose breast cancer (breast screening, mammography)?
(c)	Did you know how breast cancer is treated and where to go for the treatment?
1.2	Can you tell us about your experience with breast cancer?
(a)	When and how did you know you have cancer?
(b)	What was your first reaction when you were first diagnosed with breast cancer?
(c)	What treatment did you go through since you were diagnosed with breast cancer?
(d)	Did you do any breast screening before your breast cancer diagnosis? When did you do the last mammography?

	Section 2: Breast cancer diagnosis and distress
2.1	Tell us about any distress that you have experienced during the process of diagnosis and treatment of cancer
(a)	Emotional/psychological distress? Emotional distress during the process of treatment, change in the physical appearance
(b)	Financial distress? Distress due to impact on the financial situation.
(c)	Social isolation? (Relationship issues, heightened fear of rejection from partner loneliness)
(d)	Anxious about cancer recurrence

	Section 3: Impact of breast cancer on quality of life
3.1	How has cancer impacted your daily life and your overall quality of life?
(a)	Daily activities
(b)	Work (paid work)
(c)	Sleep (including sleep deprivation, sleep disturbances, insomnia and so on)
(d)	Cognition (memory)
(e)	Fatigue
(f)	Physical/Body image (body image was associated with mastectomies, breast reconstructive surgery, etc.)
(g)	Sexuality (Sexual disorder, discomfort)

	Section 4: Health services utilisation
4.1	Which health services are currently available to you (e.g., reproductive services, doctor's surgery and specialist services)?
4.2	Which of these services did you utilise? Tell us your experience of using these services
4.3	What health services are not available to you (e.g., reproductive services, doctor's surgery and specialist services)?
4.4	What women's health services (including reproductive health) would you like to have access to improve your health?

References

1. Australian Institute of Health and Welfare (A.I.o.H.a.W.R.). Cancer Data Australia. Available online: https://www.aihw.gov.au/getmedia/43903b67-3130-4384-8648-39c69bb684b5/Cancer-data-in-Australia.pdf.aspx?inline=true (accessed on 2 June 2021).
2. Waks, A.G.; Winer, E.P. Breast cancer treatment: A review. *JAMA* **2019**, *321*, 288–300. [CrossRef] [PubMed]
3. DeSantis, C.E.; Bray, F.; Ferlay, J.; Lortet-Tieulent, J.; Anderson, B.O.; Jemal, A. International variation in female breast cancer incidence and mortality rates. *Cancer Epidemiol. Prev. Biomark.* **2015**, *24*, 1495–1506. [CrossRef]
4. Australian Institute of Health and Welfare A.I.o.H.a.W.R. Australian Cancer Incidence and Mortality (ACIM). Available online: https://www.aihw.gov.au/reports/cancer/cancer-data-in-australia/notes (accessed on 7 May 2021).
5. Casso, D.; Buist, D.S.; Taplin, S. Quality of life of 5–10 year breast cancer survivors diagnosed between age 40 and 49. *Health Qual. Life Outcomes* **2004**, *2*, 25. [CrossRef]
6. Australian Government Department of Health (A.G.D.o.). *About the BreastScreen Australia Program*; Australian Government Department of Health: Canberra, Australia, 2021; Volume 2021.
7. Perry, L.M.; Hoerger, M.; Seibert, K.; Gerhart, J.I.; O'Mahony, S.; Duberstein, P.R. Financial strain and physical and emotional quality of life in breast cancer. *J. Pain Symptom Manag.* **2019**, *58*, 454–459. [CrossRef]
8. Campbell-Enns, H.; Woodgate, R. The psychosocial experiences of women with breast cancer across the lifespan: A systematic review protocol. *JBI Evid. Synth.* **2015**, *13*, 112–121. [CrossRef]
9. Shrout, M.R.; Renna, M.E.; Madison, A.A.; Alfano, C.M.; Povoski, S.P.; Lipari, A.M.; Agnese, D.M.; Farrar, W.B.; Carson, W.E., III; Kiecolt-Glaser, J.K. Breast cancer survivors' satisfying marriages predict better psychological and physical health: A longitudinal comparison of satisfied, dissatisfied, and unmarried women. *Psycho-Oncol.* **2021**, *30*, 699–707. [CrossRef]
10. Arora, N.K.; Gustafson, D.H.; Hawkins, R.P.; McTavish, F.; Cella, D.F.; Pingree, S.; Mendenhall, J.H.; Mahvi, D.M. Impact of surgery and chemotherapy on the quality of life of younger women with breast carcinoma: A prospective study. *Cancer Interdiscip. Int. J. Am. Cancer Soc.* **2001**, *92*, 1288–1298. [CrossRef]
11. Falk Dahl, C.A.; Reinertsen, K.V.; Nesvold, I.L.; Fosså, S.D.; Dahl, A.A. A study of body image in long-term breast cancer survivors. *Cancer* **2010**, *116*, 3549–3557. [CrossRef]
12. Abrahams, H.; Gielissen, M.; Verhagen, C.; Knoop, H. The relationship of fatigue in breast cancer survivors with quality of life and factors to address in psychological interventions: A systematic review. *Clin. Psychol. Rev.* **2018**, *63*, 1–11. [CrossRef]
13. Twombly, R. What's in a name: Who is a cancer survivor? *J. Nat. Cancer Inst.* **2004**, *96*, 1414–1415. [CrossRef] [PubMed]
14. Naik, H.; Leung, B.; Laskin, J.; McDonald, M.; Srikanthan, A.; Wu, J.; Bates, A.; Ho, C. Emotional distress and psychosocial needs in patients with breast cancer in British Columbia: Younger versus older adults. *Breast Cancer Res. Treat.* **2020**, *179*, 471–477. [CrossRef]
15. Champion, V.L.; Wagner, L.I.; Monahan, P.O.; Daggy, J.; Smith, L.; Cohee, A.; Ziner, K.W.; Haase, J.E.; Miller, K.D.; Pradhan, K. Comparison of younger and older breast cancer survivors and age-matched controls on specific and overall quality of life domains. *Cancer* **2014**, *120*, 2237–2246. [CrossRef]
16. Howard-Anderson, J.; Ganz, P.A.; Bower, J.E.; Stanton, A.L. Quality of life, fertility concerns, and behavioral health outcomes in younger breast cancer survivors: A systematic review. *J. Nat. Cancer Inst.* **2012**, *104*, 386–405. [CrossRef] [PubMed]
17. Hewitt, M.; Herdman, R.; Holland, J. Psychosocial needs of women with breast cancer. In Proceedings of the Meeting Psychosocial Needs of Women with Breast Cancer. Available online: https://www.ncbi.nlm.nih.gov/books/NBK215940/ (accessed on 10 October 2021).
18. World Health Organisation G.C.O.W.H. *Breast Cancer Fact Sheet*; World Health Organisation: Geneva, Switzerland, 2020.
19. Pope, C.; Mays, N. Qualitative research: Reaching the parts other methods cannot reach: An introduction to qualitative methods in health and health services research. *BMJ* **1995**, *311*, 42–45. [CrossRef] [PubMed]
20. Castleberry, A.; Nolen, A. Thematic analysis of qualitative research data: Is it as easy as it sounds? *Curr. Pharm. Teach. Learn.* **2018**, *10*, 807–815. [CrossRef]
21. Henselmans, I.; Helgeson, V.S.; Seltman, H.; de Vries, J.; Sanderman, R.; Ranchor, A.V. Identification and prediction of distress trajectories in the first year after a breast cancer diagnosis. *Health Psychol.* **2010**, *29*, 160–168. [CrossRef]
22. Stanton, A.L.; Ganz, P.A.; Rowland, J.H.; Meyerowitz, B.E.; Krupnick, J.L.; Sears, S.R. Promoting adjustment after treatment for cancer. *Cancer Interdiscip. Int. J. Am. Cancer Soc.* **2005**, *104*, 2608–2613. [CrossRef]
23. Henselmans, I.; Sanderman, R.; Baas, P.C.; Smink, A.; Ranchor, A.V. Personal control after a breast cancer diagnosis: Stability and adaptive value. *Psycho-Oncol. J. Psychol. Soc. Behav. Dimens. Cancer* **2009**, *18*, 104–108. [CrossRef] [PubMed]
24. Barez, M.; Blasco, T.; Fernandez-Castro, J.; Viladrich, C. A structural model of the relationships between perceived control and adaptation to illness in women with breast cancer. *J. Psychosoc. Oncol.* **2007**, *25*, 21–43. [CrossRef]
25. Gallagher, J.; Parle, M.; Cairns, D. Appraisal and psychological distress six months after diagnosis of breast cancer. *Br. J. Health Psychol.* **2002**, *7*, 365–376. [CrossRef] [PubMed]
26. Deshields, T.; Tibbs, T.; Fan, M.Y.; Taylor, M. Differences in patterns of depression after treatment for breast cancer. *Psycho-Oncol. J. Psychol. Soc. Behav. Dimens. Cancer* **2006**, *15*, 398–406. [CrossRef] [PubMed]
27. Hinnen, C.; Ranchor, A.V.; Sanderman, R.; Snijders, T.A.; Hagedoorn, M.; Coyne, J.C. Course of distress in breast cancer patients, their partners, and matched control couples. *Ann. Behav. Med.* **2008**, *36*, 141–148. [CrossRef]
28. Ward, S.E.; Viergutz, G.; Tormey, D.; DeMuth, J.; Paulen, A. Patients' reactions to completion of adjuvant breast cancer therapy. *Nurs. Res.* **1992**, *41*, 362–366. [CrossRef]

29. Oberguggenberger, A.; Meraner, V.; Sztankay, M.; Hilbert, A.; Hubalek, M.; Holzner, B.; Gamper, E.; Kemmler, G.; Baumgartner, T.; Lackinger, I. Health behavior and quality of life outcome in breast cancer survivors: Prevalence rates and predictors. *Clin. Breast Cancer* **2018**, *18*, 38–44. [CrossRef] [PubMed]
30. Pumo, V.; Milone, G.; Iacono, M.; Giuliano, S.R.; Di Mari, A.; Lopiano, C.; Bordonaro, S.; Tralongo, P. Psychological and sexual disorders in long-term breast cancer survivors. *Cancer Manag. Res.* **2012**, *4*, 61–65.
31. Davidson, J.R.; MacLean, A.W.; Brundage, M.D.; Schulze, K. Sleep disturbance in cancer patients. *Soc. Sci. Med.* **2002**, *54*, 1309–1321. [CrossRef]
32. Beck, S.L.; Berger, A.M.; Barsevick, A.M.; Wong, B.; Stewart, K.A.; Dudley, W.N. Sleep quality after initial chemotherapy for breast cancer. *Support. Care Cancer* **2010**, *18*, 679–689. [CrossRef]
33. Bower, J.E.; Ganz, P.A.; Desmond, K.A.; Bernaards, C.; Rowland, J.H.; Meyerowitz, B.E.; Belin, T.R. Fatigue in long-term breast carcinoma survivors: A longitudinal investigation. *Cancer* **2006**, *106*, 751–758. [CrossRef]
34. Collins, B.; Mackenzie, J.; Stewart, A.; Bielajew, C.; Verma, S. Cognitive effects of hormonal therapy in early stage breast cancer patients: A prospective study. *Psycho-Oncol. J. Psychol. Soc. Behav. Dimens. Cancer* **2009**, *18*, 811–821. [CrossRef]
35. Nelson, W.L.; Suls, J. New approaches to understand cognitive changes associated with chemotherapy for non-central nervous system tumors. *J. Pain Symptom Manag.* **2013**, *46*, 707–721. [CrossRef]
36. Coyne, E.; Wollin, J.; Creedy, D.K. Exploration of the family's role and strengths after a young woman is diagnosed with breast cancer: Views of women and their families. *Eur. J. Oncol. Nurs.* **2012**, *16*, 124–130. [CrossRef] [PubMed]
37. Halkett, G.; Arbon, P.; Scutter, S.; Borg, M. The role of the breast care nurse during treatment for early breast cancer: The patient's perspective. *Contemp. Nurse* **2006**, *23*, 46–57. [CrossRef] [PubMed]
38. Keesing, S.; Rosenwax, L.; McNamara, B. A dyadic approach to understanding the impact of breast cancer on relationships between partners during early survivorship. *BMC Women's Health* **2016**, *16*, 57. [CrossRef]
39. Perz, J.; Ussher, J.; Gilbert, E. Loss, uncertainty, or acceptance: Subjective experience of changes to fertility after breast cancer. *Eur. J. Cancer Care* **2014**, *23*, 514–522. [CrossRef] [PubMed]
40. Spence, D.; Morstyn, L.; Wells, K. The support and information needs of women with secondary breast cancer. *Breast Cancer Netw. Aust.* 2015. Available online: https://www.bcna.org.au/media/2936/bcn1166-sbc-report-2015.pdf (accessed on 10 October 2021).
41. Mehnert, A. Employment and work-related issues in cancer survivors. *Crit. Rev. Oncol. Hematol.* **2011**, *77*, 109–130. [CrossRef] [PubMed]

Case Report

Intervention of Coordination by Liaison Nurse Where Ward Staff Struggled to Establish a Therapeutic Relationship with a Patient Because of Failure to Recognize Delirium: A Case Study

Yuri Nakai [1], Yusuke Nitta [2,*] and Reiko Hashimoto [2]

1. Faculty of Nursing, University of Kochi, 2751-1 Ike, Kochi City 780-8515, Japan; nakai_yuri@cc.u-kochi.ac.jp
2. Department of Neuropsychiatry, Kanazawa Medical University, 1-1 Uchinada, Kahoku 920-0265, Japan; reipon@kanazawa-med.ac.jp
* Correspondence: nta-ysk@kanazawa-med.ac.jp; Tel.: +81-76-286-2211 (ext. 3437)

Abstract: In this case study, ward staff found it difficult to establish a therapeutic relationship with a patient with advanced gastric cancer because they misdiagnosed delirium as a psychogenic reaction to the cancer diagnosis. This article reports on the process and effects of intervention by a liaison nurse. The liaison nurse recognized the misdiagnosis and approached the ward staff via a psychiatrist-led team. This enabled rapid revision of the treatment policy. The liaison nurse contributed to the continuation of treatment by enabling the ward staff and patient to understand each other better and to collaborate to build a relationship and control the patient's mental health symptoms, including attention disorder and excessive demands. The patient and family had different views on discharge because of the patient's mental health issues. The liaison nurse encouraged the ward staff to inform the family caregiver about the patient's medical condition, the expected future course of the disease, and likely symptoms, and provide appropriate professional services. This enabled the patient to be discharged in line with their wishes. This case highlights the role of the liaison nurse in coordinating care and helping ward staff to recognize symptoms and provide appropriate care and support for patients and their families.

Keywords: delirium; liaison nurse; misrecognition of delirium; coordination

1. Introduction

Delirium is caused by a range of factors such as the presence of predisposing conditions, including cognitive impairment, severe illness, visual impairment, drug therapy, and hospitalization [1]. When delirium develops during treatment, it interrupts the treatment and increases the risk of complications and further functional deterioration. It is associated with adverse events such as confusion and falls in hospitalized patients [2], and self-extraction of the infusion line [3]. This may mean that the length of hospital stay is extended, and labor costs and material costs for the stay are both increased [4]. This can also increase mortality [5]. The etiology of delirium is unknown, but prophylactic nursing interventions may be an efficient and cost-effective solution [6]. Careful observation and intervention by nurses are important to avoid the adverse consequences of delirium, allow patients to receive the desired treatment, and return to their daily lives.

The prevalence of delirium in cancer patients increases toward the end of life [7]. Delirium is a common psychiatric complication in cancer patients, but it is often not accurately recognized. In one study of psychiatric examinations of cancer patients, doctors were distracted by symptoms such as pain and missed the diagnosis of delirium in 46% of patients [8]. Overall, 61% of patients referred to palliative care had delirium overlooked by the primary referral team [9]. Approximately 50% of the primary teams of patients referred to liaison services for reasons other than delirium were unaware of the delirium [10]. In particular, delirium is prone to be unrecognized in younger cancer patients [11]. The symptoms of delirium are diverse and appear irregularly. Patients with delirium may also try to address or hide agitation, apathy, emotional instability, and disorientation [12]. If treatment continues without the presence of delirium being recognized, it will have less or no therapeutic effect. Misdiagnosis can also lengthen the period in which nurses have difficulty responding to the patient, which can have effects on the whole ward. The nurses and medical staff who directly respond to patients' abuse and excessive demands are especially likely to experience serious psychological distress and stress. Nurses have the most frequent and closest contact with patients and play an important role in caring for and comforting delirium patients. It is therefore very important to be aware of and minimize their needs and stress [13]. Nurses and medical staff may also develop negative feelings toward patients with unrecognized delirium, which hinders the proper treatment and care for these patients. Early recognition of delirium, identification of possible causes, and provision of knowledgeable care will improve the quality and outcome of patient care [1,14]. If a nurse or other member of staff may have failed to recognize delirium, rapid intervention is needed to address the situation and reorient both patient and staff to appropriate treatment and care. Certified nurse specialists (CNS) in Japan are nurses who participate in clinical practice, consultation, coordination of activities, ethical management, education, and research [15]. These nurses are responsible for guiding staff in difficult situations, identifying learning needs, and highlighting the right approach [16]. They can therefore improve outcomes for patients.

In the case reported here, nurses and medical staff failed to recognize a variety of psychological symptoms caused by delirium in a gastric cancer patient. Instead, they believed that these were psychogenic reactions associated with the patient's recent diagnosis of advanced gastric cancer. It was therefore difficult for the nurses to establish a therapeutic relationship with the patient. The purpose of this study is to report on the process and effects of coordination and intervention by the CNS who was part of the liaison team. This may help to improve best practice for delirium cases in younger cancer patients.

2. Case Presentation
2.1. Terminology
2.1.1. Liaison Team

The liaison team in Japan is a team of three or more people, including a psychiatrist, a nurse with more than 3 years of experience in psychiatry, and a medical professional with more than 3 years of experience in psychiatry. Medical professionals include pharmacists, occupational therapists, mental health social workers, and certified psychologists. The liaison team treats and cares for mental health symptoms and psychological problems of hospitalized patients and their families, using specialized skills from a physical, mental, and social perspective. The team aims to improve the mental health of patients and their families. It also supports the physical and mental health of staff involved in treatment, improves their motivation to work, and prevents them from burning out [17,18].

2.1.2. Certified Nurse Specialist (CNS)

A certified nurse specialist is a nurse who has completed the certified nurse specialist education course at a Japanese graduate school and has passed the certified nurse specialist certification examination. As of February 2022, there are 14 specialist fields, including cancer nursing, psychiatric mental health nursing, and community health nursing. CNSs have six key roles: practice, consultation, coordination, ethical coordination, education, and research [19].

2.2. Case Information

This case report describes a woman in her 40s. She works as a salesperson, has never been married, and lives alone. Her parents are dead. Her family caregiver is her younger brother. Her only medical history is an oral treatment for bronchial asthma. She has no history of psychiatric treatment.

2.3. Clinical Findings

In June 20XX, the patient complained of an enlarged feeling in her abdomen and was diagnosed with advanced gastric cancer (stage IV). She was admitted to medical oncology on July 18. After admission, she was informed that her prognosis was 1 year. She chose to receive chemotherapy and started anticancer drugs (TS1 + cisplatin) (SP therapy) on July 20th. The second cycle was carried out on 10 August. From 15 August, she started frequent refusal of treatment and examinations and behaved aggressively toward the ward staff. On the night of 30 August, the patient's words and actions became uncoordinated and communication became difficult. Her dissatisfaction, anger, and shouting worsened. The patient's symptoms and ward staff behavior by stage of medical treatment are shown below.

1. 30 August–14 September

After August 10th, the patient was reported as developing an intimidating attitude and emotional instability, making excessive demands on the nurses, having a silly smile, and being silent and immobile. The ward staff decided that these symptoms were a psychogenic reaction to the news that the cancer was advanced. They, therefore, responded without complaint to the patient's demands and requests.

2. 15 September–10 October

The patient was prescribed an antipsychotic drug, and her anger disappeared, but the irritability remained. The psychological burden on the ward staff was heavy, and they continued to struggle to deal with the patient. The patient started to show overactivity, attention dysfunction, excessive demands, and frequent family phone calls. These seem to have been triggered by spending nights away from the ward, and the resumption of the therapy. The psychological burden on the ward staff, therefore, became even higher, and they began to complain to the head nurse that it was difficult to deal with this patient on a general ward.

3. 11 October–1 November

After three cycles of SP therapy, the patient showed attention dysfunction and garrulity, but wanted to be discharged to the community and live alone. The ward staff decided that she would be able to do this by using social resources such as home-visit nursing. However, her family caregiver thought it would be difficult for her to live alone because of her symptoms. He was also worried that if the patient's condition worsened or suddenly changed, treatment would be delayed. There was therefore a conflict of opinion about discharge between the patient and her family caregiver. The ward staff respected the views of the family caregiver rather than those of the patient and suggested that the patient should give up the idea of living alone.

2.4. Timeline

The phase-by-phase medical conditions and the liaison nurse's interventions are shown below.

The need for the liaison nurse to intervene, and the nurse's actions, were classified into Phases 1, 2, and 3 by treatment and date. Figure 1 shows the patient's physical and psychotic symptoms, blood test values, and treatments by phase.

		Phase 1 8/30–9/14		Phase 2 9/15–10/10		Phase 3 10/11–11/1		
Duration of hospitalization	7/18 Admission			9/15 O	10/4–6 O	10/11 Family caregiver came	10/21 O	11/1 Discharge
				(O : Overnight stay at home)				
Chemotherapy	7/20 SP therapy: 1	8/10 SP therapy: 2		9/20 SP therapy: 3		10/18 SP therapy: 4		
Physical symptoms	Ascites Edema Sluggishness Constipation	Nausea Taste disorders Constipation Diarrhea		Taste disorders Edema		Taste disorders		
Hb (g/dl)	13.2	11.4	9.4	9.4		9.1	10.1	
CRP (mg/dl)	0.11	0.58	7.5	0.10		0.25	0.04	
Na (mEq/l)	139	140	132	139		142	142	
Cr (mg/dl)	0.67	0.51	0.49	0.38		0.51	0.53	
Alb (g/dl)	3.7	3.2	1.8	3.1		2.8	3.7	
Psychiatric symptoms		Coercive and excessive demands, silly smile, silence, immobility	Irritability, garrulity, overactivity, hyperthymia	Garrulity, overactivity, hyperthymia		Garrulity		
			Attention disorder (repeating the same story, inability to concentrate on the task)					
			Difficulty falling asleep					
Medication			↑ Haloperidol 2.5mg			Valproic acid 400mg	200mg	
			Quetiapine 25mg 50mg	Olanzapine 5mg				

Figure 1. Physical and psychotic symptoms by phase, blood test values, and treatment.

2.5. Therapeutic Interventions

2.5.1. Interventions of the Liaison Nurse with Ward Staff: Phase 1

Coordination by Liaison Nurse in Phase 1

The liaison nurse held a conference with the liaison team and ward staff to correct the failure to recognize delirium. At the conference, the liaison nurse explained that the patient's psychological symptoms may be caused by delirium related to the chemotherapy, rather than a psychogenic reaction to her diagnosis. The team then clarified the role of each group of staff in supporting patients with delirium, to help to rebuild the support relationship between the patient and ward staff. Physical management of the patient was the responsibility of the doctor in charge of cancer treatment, nurses and physiotherapists should provide a non-pharmaceutical response to paralysis, and the liaison team would manage the mental health of the patient and support the mental health of ward staff (Table 1).

Table 1. Patient's delirium symptoms in Phase 1, state of ward staff, and liaison nurse intervention needs.

State of Patient	State of Ward Staff	Assessment of Intervention Needs
The patient rapidly developed an intimidating attitude, emotional instability, silly smile, silence, and immobility, and started making excessive demands on the nurses.	Staff decided that the patient's psychological symptoms were a psychogenic reaction to the news of the cancer. The staff gradually found it more difficult to respond and became more psychologically burdened, and more negative about the patient.	It was difficult for the staff to deal with the patient's mental health issues because they had failed to recognize that she was experiencing delirium.

2.5.2. Education on How to Deal with Attention Disorders, Rebuilding the Therapeutic Relationship between Patients and Ward Staff: Phase 2

Coordination by Liaison Nurse in Phase 2

The liaison nurse suggested how to respond to the concern from the ward staff that resuming SP therapy would worsen the patient's psychological symptoms. The team worked with the patient and nurses to enable certified psychologists to conduct an evaluation of the patient's condition using the Japanese version of the Young Mania Rating Scale (YMRS-J) and to consider countermeasures. The liaison nurse assisted in communication about countermeasures to make it easier for the patient and nurses to talk about their concerns. The agreed measures were as follows: (1) the patient should self-check her mental condition; (2) the patient should inform nurses if she becomes aware of any changes in her mental state; (3) nurses should carefully observe any changes in the patient's mental state; (4) if either the patient or nurses noticed changes in the patient's mental state, they should discuss this together and consider how to deal with it, and (5) the nurse in charge should inform all ward staff about the coping method jointly decided by the patient and the nurse in charge to provide a unified response (Table 2).

Table 2. Patient's delirium symptoms in Phase 2, state of ward staff, and liaison nurse intervention needs.

State of Patient	State of Ward Staff	Assessment of Intervention Needs
Irritability, attention disorders, and overactivity remained, and the psychological symptoms worsened because of the resumption of SP therapy. Self-care ability therefore declined.	The ward staff decided that it would be difficult to deal with the mental symptoms because of the resumption of SP therapy. They therefore found it difficult to continue treatment of the patient on the general ward.	Support to manage the situation where the ward staff judged that it was difficult to respond to the patient on the general ward.

After this discussion, the nurse in charge commented:

"I didn't point out her psychological symptoms to the patient because I was afraid that doing so would worsen her intimidating attitude, emotional instability, and excessive demands." She added,

"I learned that the practice of sharing psychological symptoms with patients and considering countermeasures can be an option as an intervention method."

2.5.3. Managing a Conflict of Views about the Patient's Discharge from the Hospital: Phase 3

Coordination by Liaison Nurse in Phase 3

The liaison nurse suggested that the ward staff should find out more about the background behind the family caregiver's opposition to the patient's discharge to the community. She suggested the following three actions: (1) ward staff should try to understand the family caregiver's concerns; (2) ward staff should identify the reason for concerns and intervene to reduce the family caregiver's anxiety, and (3) ward staff should guarantee to the family caregiver that the hospital would continue to provide treatment support, psychiatric support, and living support to help the patient use social resources even after she was discharged to the community (Table 3).

Table 3. Patient's delirium symptoms in Phase 3, state of ward staff, and liaison nurse intervention needs.

State of Patient	State of Ward Staff	Assessment of Intervention Needs
The attention disorder and garrulity remained, but the patient expressed her intention of leaving the hospital to live alone in the community.	The ward staff decided that it was possible for the patient to live alone by using social resources such as home-visit nursing. However, the family caregiver was concerned about changes in the patient's personality, her attention disorder and residual garrulity, and the potential for sudden changes in her illness. He suggested that it would be difficult for her to live alone. The ward staff supported this view once expressed.	The liaison nurse needed to manage the conflict of views about the patient's discharge from the hospital. This was particularly important given the small amount of time left for her to live, and the potential that her wishes might not be respected.

3. Discussion

In cases where the liaison nurse finds an unrecognized patient with dementia in the ward, a patient has a mental health problem, (e.g., attention disorder or excessive demands) due to dementia caused by chemotherapy and has an issue with the discharge destination, or there is a conflict of intention between the patient and family caregiver regarding the discharge destination, the liaison nurse will coordinate interventions as described below.

Delirium is the most common complication in patients with advanced cancer. However, it is often difficult to identify, which leads to improper management [20]. Delirium in younger patients in particular may be missed because of the lack of disorientation [21]. The patient in this case study showed emotional instability and an intimidating attitude toward the nurses. The patient was in her 40s and the ward staff may have failed to recognize her delirium because she had no symptoms of disorientation. If someone identifies a patient with delirium-induced psychological symptoms that have not previously been recognized, it is important to provide a correct diagnosis as soon as possible, so that appropriate treatment or care can be provided. In this case, the correction using a team approach centered on the liaison psychiatrist helped the ward staff to quickly correct the misrecognition. It seems likely that ward staff will find it easier to accept a correction from the liaison team as a whole, rather than the liaison nurse alone. We suggest that this approach enabled the misrecognition to be corrected promptly. The ward staff and liaison team then correctly diagnosed the situation and worked together to solve the problem.

It is probable that the ward staff had high levels of negative feelings toward the patient because of the stress placed on them by the patient's intimidating attitude and excessive demands. Nurses should not rush to diagnose a patient with delirium, but should be aware that patients may have this condition [22]. Cases of hypomanic symptoms have been reported during S1 and cisplatin therapy for patients with gastric cancer [23], but it is not common. It is, therefore, possible that the staff on this ward were unfamiliar with psychological symptoms and did not appreciate the possibility of delirium. However, they did recognize the association with the SP therapy and suggested that, if the symptoms recurred on further treatment, it would be difficult for them to manage. The liaison nurse found that the ward staff felt responsible for managing all the patient's psychological symptoms when they occurred on the ward. The liaison nurse, therefore, contributed to the continuation of treatment by observing the mental health symptoms of the ward staff and working with the patient to enable her to self-check her own symptoms.

In Phase 3, the patient and family caregiver disagreed about discharge. The patient wanted to be discharged to the community, but the family caregiver thought this would be difficult because of the patient's complex psychological symptoms. Ward staff supported the family caregiver's view. This is considered inappropriate in this case because they had initially supported discharge and because of the patient's short life expectancy. It is important to provide information and involve family caregivers when older people are discharged from the hospital [24]. Family caregivers involved in discharge planning are more likely to accept the role of providing post-discharge care [25]. In this case, the family caregiver's view suggests that they were given little information and not involved in the discharge planning. A previous study found that failure to discharge a COPD patient because of a bureaucratic organizational workflow may not be in the patient's best interests [26]. In this case, it is possible that ward staff felt that the family caregiver's opposition to the patient's discharge to the community would make the process harder. This suggests that the organization as a whole may not be focused on the best interests of the patient. Other studies have noted that the actions of liaison nurses in the discharge process, and especially coordinating with a specialist on behalf of the patient, help to continue care after discharge [27]. In this case, the liaison nurse's intervention to prompt the ward staff to provide more information to the family caregiver may have contributed to discharge, in line with the patient's wishes. The liaison nurse asked the ward staff to explain to the family caregiver about the changes in the patient's personality, and provide more information about the attention disorder, and how it affected behavior. The liaison team also asked the ward staff to arrange for treatment and home-based services for the patient after she was discharged. This support included home-visit nursing services, confirmed contact information in an emergency, a continuous support system by the hospital, and access to a consultation desk for family caregivers. In this case, the liaison nurse helped the ward staff to understand the challenges, and also evaluated their direct care and support to the patient and family.

This case report has some limitations. First, it is a report of a single case and cannot be generalized. Second, the classification of Phases 1–3 is based on our assessment of the patient's treatment stage, and not on existing theories or protocols. Third, this paper focused on the intervention of the liaison nurse and its effects; however, the intervention of the liaison team as a whole may also have influenced the effects. Despite these limitations, this case report provides useful information for the practice of liaison nurses working with staff who have difficulty responding to changes in personality and diverse psychological symptoms in patients with advanced cancer.

4. Conclusions

If a liaison nurse discovers a patient with delirium that has not been recognized on the ward, we recommend that the mistake is pointed out by the whole liaison team, led by liaison psychiatrists. This is because ward staff may be offended by having their mistake highlighted by another nurse, and may not be prepared to consider the possibility of delirium. For mental health problems such as attention disorder and excessive demands caused by delirium arising from chemotherapy, the liaison nurse should support the ward staff and patient to observe each other's psychological symptoms and work together to build a relationship that can control the symptoms. To enable patients with advanced cancer to make their own decisions about their lives, the liaison nurse needs to help the ward staff to provide family caregivers with information about the medical condition, its expected future course and symptoms, and professional services that are available to help.

Author Contributions: Y.N. (Yuri Nakai) and Y.N. (Yusuke Nitta); methodology, Y.N. (Yuri Nakai) and Y.N. (Yusuke Nitta); formal analysis, Y.N. (Yuri Nakai), Y.N. (Yusuke Nitta) and R.H.; investigation, Y.N. (Yuri Nakai), Y.N. (Yusuke Nitta) and R.H.; resources, Y.N. (Yuri Nakai), Y.N. (Yusuke Nitta) and R.H.; data curation, Y.N. (Yuri Nakai); writing—original draft preparation, Y.N. (Yuri Nakai), Y.N. (Yusuke Nitta) and R.H.; writing—review and editing, Y.N. (Yuri Nakai) and Y.N. (Yusuke Nitta); visualization, Y.N. (Yusuke Nitta); supervision. All authors have read and agreed to the published version of the manuscript.

Funding: This research received no external funding.

Institutional Review Board Statement: This research was conducted in accordance with the Declaration of Helsinki, 1995 (as revised in Seoul, 2008) and carried out with the consent of the medical research ethics review committees at the Kanazawa Medical University Hospitals (No. H266).

Informed Consent Statement: Informed consent was obtained from the patient involved in the case study.

Data Availability Statement: Not applicable.

Acknowledgments: We thank Melissa Leffler for editing a draft of this manuscript.

Conflicts of Interest: The authors declare no conflict of interest.

References

1. Inouye, S.K.; Bogardus, S.T.; Charpentier, P.A.; Leo-Summers, L.; Acampora, D.; Holford, T.R.; Cooney, L.M. A Multicomponent Intervention to Prevent Delirium in Hospitalized Older Patients. *N. Engl. J. Med.* **1999**, *340*, 669–676. [CrossRef] [PubMed]
2. Lakatos, B.E.; Capasso, V.; Mitchell, M.T.; Kilroy, S.M.; Lussier-Cushing, M.; Sumner, L.; Repper-Delisi, J.; Kelleher, E.P.; Delisle, L.A.; Cruz, C.; et al. Falls in the General Hospital: Association With Delirium, Advanced Age, and Specific Surgical Procedures. *Psychosomatics* **2009**, *50*, 218–226. [CrossRef] [PubMed]
3. Dubois, M.-J.; Bergeron, N.; Dumont, M.; Dial, S.; Skrobik, Y. Delirium in an Intensive Care Unit: A Study of Risk Factors. *Intensive Care Med.* **2001**, *27*, 1297–1304. [CrossRef] [PubMed]
4. Weinrebe, W.; Johannsdottir, E.; Karaman, M.; Füsgen, I. What Does Delirium Cost? *Z. Gerontol. Geriat.* **2016**, *49*, 52–58. [CrossRef] [PubMed]
5. Witlox, J.; Eurelings, L.S.M.; de Jonghe, J.F.M.; Kalisvaart, K.J.; Eikelenboom, P.; van Gool, W.A. Delirium in Elderly Patients and the Risk of Postdischarge Mortality, Institutionalization, and Dementia: A Meta-Analysis. *JAMA* **2010**, *304*, 443–451. [CrossRef]
6. Méndez-Martínez, C.; Fernández-Martínez, M.N.; García-Suárez, M.; Martínez-Isasi, S.; Fernández-Fernández, J.A.; Fernández-García, D. Related Factors and Treatment of Postoperative Delirium in Old Adult Patients: An Integrative Review. *Healthcare* **2021**, *9*, 1103. [CrossRef]
7. Caraceni, A. Drug-Associated Delirium in Cancer Patients. *Eur. J. Cancer Suppl.* **2013**, *11*, 233–240. [CrossRef]
8. Kishi, Y.; Kato, M.; Okuyama, T.; Hosaka, T.; Mikami, K.; Meller, W.; Thurber, S.; Kathol, R. Delirium: Patient Characteristics That Predict a Missed Diagnosis at Psychiatric Consultation. *Gen. Hosp. Psychiatry* **2007**, *29*, 442–445. [CrossRef]
9. de la Cruz, M.; Fan, J.; Yennu, S.; Tanco, K.; Shin, S.; Wu, J.; Liu, D.; Bruera, E. The Frequency of Missed Delirium in Patients Referred to Palliative Care in a Comprehensive Cancer Center. *Support Care Cancer* **2015**, *23*, 2427–2433. [CrossRef]
10. Mittal, D.; Majithia, D.; Kennedy, R.; Rhudy, J. Differences in Characteristics and Outcome of Delirium as Based on Referral Patterns. *Psychosomatics* **2006**, *47*, 367–375. [CrossRef]
11. Wada, T.; Wada, M.; Wada, M.; Onishi, H. Characteristics, interventions, and outcomes of misdiagnosed delirium in cancer patients. *Palliat. Supportive Care* **2010**, *8*, 125–131. [CrossRef] [PubMed]
12. Kang, J.H.; Shin, S.H.; Bruera, E. Comprehensive Approaches to Managing Delirium in Patients with Advanced Cancer. *Cancer Treat. Rev.* **2013**, *39*, 105–112. [CrossRef]
13. O'Malley, G.; Leonard, M.; Meagher, D.; O'Keeffe, S.T. The Delirium Experience: A Review. *J. Psychosom. Res.* **2008**, *65*, 223–228. [CrossRef]
14. Boot, R. Delirium: A Review of the Nurses Role in the Intensive Care Unit. *Intensive Crit. Care Nurs.* **2012**, *28*, 185–189. [CrossRef] [PubMed]
15. Kitajima, M.; Miyata, C.; Tamura, K.; Kinoshita, A.; Arai, H. Factors associated with the job satisfaction of certified nurses and nurse specialists in cancer care in Japan: Analysis based on the Basic Plan to Promote Cancer Control Programs. *PLoS ONE* **2020**, *15*, e0232336. [CrossRef] [PubMed]
16. LaSala, C.A.; Connors, P.M.; Pedro, J.T.; Phipps, M. The Role of the Clinical Nurse Specialist in Promoting Evidence-Based Practice and Effecting Positive Patient Outcomes. *J. Contin. Educ. Nurs.* **2007**, *38*, 262–270. [CrossRef]
17. Psychiatric Medicine (2011_11_2) Ministry of Health, Labour and Welfare (Japanese). Available online: https://www.mhlw.go.jp/stf/shingi/2r9852000001trya-att/2r9852000001ts1s.pdf (accessed on 22 May 2022).
18. Koichi, M.; Kazuko, N.; Kawori, I.; Yukihiro, T.; Keiko, M. Practice of Psychiatry Liaison Teams at General Hospitals without a Specialized Psychiatry Inpatient Unit (Japanese). *Jpn. J. Gen. Hosp. Psychiatry* **2013**, *25*, 130–143. [CrossRef]
19. Japan Nursing Association Qualification Certification System, Japan Nursing Association (Japanese). Available online: https://nintei.nurse.or.jp/nursing/qualification/cns (accessed on 22 May 2022).
20. Centeno, C.; Sanz, Á.; Bruera, E. Delirium in Advanced Cancer Patients. *Palliat. Med.* **2004**, *18*, 184–194. [CrossRef]
21. Swigart, S.E.; Kishi, Y.; Thurber, S.; Kathol, R.G.; Meller, W.H. Misdiagnosed Delirium in Patient Referrals to a University-Based Hospital Psychiatry Department. *Psychosomatics* **2008**, *49*, 104–108. [CrossRef]
22. Ozga, D.; Krupa, S.; Witt, P.; Mędrzycka-Dąbrowska, W. Nursing Interventions to Prevent Delirium in Critically Ill Patients in the Intensive Care Unit during the COVID19 Pandemic—Narrative Overview. *Healthcare* **2020**, *8*, 578. [CrossRef]
23. Matsunaga, M.; Onishi, H.; Ishida, M.; Miwa, K.; Araki, K.; Kaneta, T.; Sunakawa, Y.; Nakayama, H.; Shimada, K.; Noguchi, T.; et al. Hypomanic Episode During Recurrent Gastric Cancer Treatment: Report of a Rare Case and Literature Review. *Jpn. J. Clin. Oncol.* **2012**, *42*, 961–964. [CrossRef] [PubMed]
24. Bull, M.J.; Roberts, J. Components of a Proper Hospital Discharge for Elders. *J. Adv. Nurs.* **2001**, *35*, 571–581. [CrossRef] [PubMed]
25. Bull, M.J.; Hansen, H.E.; Gross, C.R. Differences in Family Caregiver Outcomes by Their Level of Involvement in Discharge Planning. *Appl. Nurs. Res.* **2000**, *13*, 76–82. [CrossRef]

26. Nnate, D.A.; Barber, D.; Abaraogu, U.O. Discharge Plan to Promote Patient Safety and Shared Decision Making by a Multidisciplinary Team of Healthcare Professionals in a Respiratory Unit. *Nurs. Rep.* **2021**, *11*, 590–599. [CrossRef] [PubMed]
27. Aued, G.K.; Bernardino, E.; Lapierre, J.; Dallaire, C. Liaison Nurse Activities at Hospital Discharge: A Strategy for Continuity of Care. *Rev. Lat.-Am. Enferm.* **2019**, *27*, e3162. [CrossRef]

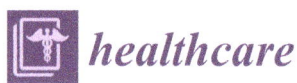
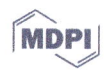

Article

Psychosocial Intervention Cultural Adaptation for Latinx Patients and Caregivers Coping with Advanced Cancer

Normarie Torres-Blasco [1,*], Rosario Costas-Muñiz [2], Lianel Rosario [1], Laura Porter [3], Keishliany Suárez [1], Cristina Peña-Vargas [1], Yoamy Toro-Morales [1], Megan Shen [4], William Breitbart [2] and Eida M. Castro-Figueroa [1]

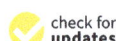

Citation: Torres-Blasco, N.; Costas-Muñiz, R.; Rosario, L.; Porter, L.; Suárez, K.; Peña-Vargas, C.; Toro-Morales, Y.; Shen, M.; Breitbart, W.; Castro-Figueroa, E.M. Psychosocial Intervention Cultural Adaptation for Latinx Patients and Caregivers Coping with Advanced Cancer. *Healthcare* 2022, 10, 1243. https://doi.org/10.3390/healthcare10071243

Academic Editor: Margaret Fitch

Received: 18 April 2022
Accepted: 29 June 2022
Published: 4 July 2022

Publisher's Note: MDPI stays neutral with regard to jurisdictional claims in published maps and institutional affiliations.

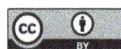

Copyright: © 2022 by the authors. Licensee MDPI, Basel, Switzerland. This article is an open access article distributed under the terms and conditions of the Creative Commons Attribution (CC BY) license (https://creativecommons.org/licenses/by/4.0/).

[1] School of Behavioral and Brain Sciences, Ponce Health Science University, Ponce, PR 00717, USA; lrosario21@stu.psm.edu (L.R.); ksuarez21@stu.psm.edu (K.S.); cpena@psm.edu (C.P.-V.); ytoro19@stu.psm.edu (Y.T.-M.); ecastro@psm.edu (E.M.C.-F.)
[2] Memorial Sloan-Kettering Cancer Center, Department of Psychiatry & Behavioral Sciences, New York, NY 10065, USA; costasmr@mskcc.org (R.C.-M.); breitbartw@mskcc.org (W.B.)
[3] Department of Psychiatry & Behavioral Sciences, Duke University Medical Center, Durham, NC 27708, USA; laura.porter@duke.edu
[4] Fred Hutchinson Cancer Center, Clinical Research Division, Seattle, WA 98109, USA; mshen2@fredhutch.org
* Correspondence: normarietorres@psm.edu

Abstract: Latinx advanced cancer patients and caregivers are less likely to have adequate access to culturally congruent psychosocial interventions. Culturally relevant and adapted interventions are more effective within minority groups. We obtained patients' and caregivers' initial evaluations of the Caregivers–Patients Support to Latinx coping with advanced-cancer (CASA) protocol. A qualitative study was conducted, and an acceptance questionnaire and semi-structured interviews were conducted to culturally adapt the psychosocial intervention for Latinx coping with cancer. The semi-structured interview described and demonstrated intervention components and elicited feedback about each one. Latinx advanced cancer patients (Stage III and IV) and caregivers (n = 14 each) completed the acceptance survey, and N = 7 each completed semi-structured interviews. A total of 12 of the 14 patients and caregivers (85.7%) reported high acceptance of the goals and purposes of the intervention protocol. They also reported willingness to daily use of the content of the intervention components: Communication Skills, the Willingness of Meaning, Life has Meaning, Freedom of Will, Identity, Creative Sources of Meaning, and Homework. Most of the participants reported high acceptance (n = 9) of integrating family caregivers into therapy and the high acceptance (n = 10) of the length of the 4-session intervention.

Keywords: Latinx; family; meaning; communication; coping with advanced cancer

1. Introduction

Adapting and developing culturally sensitive interventions is needed for Latinx families coping with advanced cancer (stage III or IV) [1–3]. Latinx patients coping with cancer have reported the need to include cultural values such as family and spirituality [4,5]. Family is a core value in the Latinx community and may facilitate the caring process for this group's advanced cancer patients [6–8]. The inclusion of Latinx values is especially essential when evidence suggests that working with spirituality and family needs (e.g., communication) could improve psychological symptoms [6–8].

Including cultural values is critical to developing a culturally sensitive intervention. The adaptation of culturally sensitive interventions is more effective towards the specific culture, rather than non-adapted interventions [9]. The cultural adaptation of evidence-based interventions (e.g., meaning-centered psychotherapy and couple communication training skills) is feasible and acceptable for ethnic minority groups [9–12]. Meta-analytic evidence suggests that culturally adapted interventions targeting a specific cultural group (e.g., Puerto Ricans as part of the Latinx community) are four times more effective than those provided to groups containing various cultural backgrounds [12].

Most literature among advanced cancer patients has been developed for white patients and not adapted for Latinx patients and caregivers. Cultural adaptation of interventions designed to support advanced cancer patients and their families is a novel approach that may benefit both patients and caregivers [9–12] coping with advanced cancer. An intervention for advanced Latinx cancer patients and caregivers should consider cultural values that may affect the end-of-life process [13]. This study aimed to obtain advanced cancer patients' and caregivers' initial evaluations of a protocol titled: Caregivers–Patients Support to Latinx coping advanced-cancer (CASA). In this brief report, the study team included results from interviews conducted with patients and caregivers to help adjust and refine the protocol.

2. Method

The present study consisted of qualitative analyses for the semi-structured interview, alongside descriptive statistics for the demographic and acceptance questionnaire. The Ponce Research Institute Institutional Review Board (IRB), with the permission of the oncology clinic, approved all study procedures. Participants were recruited from an oncology clinic in southern Puerto Rico referred by the nurse or oncologist. Potential participants were introduced to the study by an IRB-approved introductory letter. This was followed by an in-person research staff meeting with participants to provide information, answer questions, and administer the Distress Thermometer to determine eligibility. The inclusion criteria for both patients and caregivers was a score > 3 on the Distress Thermometer. Those eligible and interested completed an informed consent form. A call was scheduled for those who consented to complete the questionnaire and interview. Patients and caregivers each received USD 30 for completing the interview and volunteering their time and effort. An a priori sample size of 14 participants was selected based on recommendations for qualitative studies of this nature [14,15].

The team collected demographic information and acceptance questionnaire responses from patients and caregivers separately (14 patients and 14 caregivers) and then conducted a one-time 45 min semi-structured interview (NTB) that introduced information about the intervention to participants and elicited their feedback using a standardized interview guide. Patients and caregivers were interviewed separately so their responses would not be affected. The interviewer described and provided examples of intervention components (see Table 1) and elicited feedback about each intervention component and format in the semi-structured interview. Participants were also asked about their preferred mode of intervention delivery. Interviews were audio-recorded and then transcribed. The study team reviewed the recordings and transcriptions and analyzed them using thematic content coding [14,15].

The measures used in this project are a demographic questionnaire, an acceptance questionnaire, and a semi-structured interview. The demographic questionnaire includes questions regarding biological sex, age, employment, years of school completed, marital status, insurance, annual income, type of cancer, and caregiver relationship with the patient. The acceptance questionnaire comprised 34 questions assessing the acceptance of the goals and concepts of meaning-centered psychotherapy (MCP, 16 items), couples communication skills training (CCST, 8 items), and the feasibility of the goals and therapeutic methods (10 items) of MCP and CCST. The acceptance questions assess the importance of the concepts and goals. The feasibility questions assess the likelihood of participating in a psychotherapy intervention. The semi-structured interview describes the CASA intervention content (Table 1) and includes five sections: (1) purpose and goals; (2) intervention content—MCP and CCST; (3) homework; (4) other possible topics for discussion; and (5) intervention format.

Table 1. Caregivers–Patients Support to Latinx coping advanced-cancer" (CASA) content presented in the interview. The X indicate the inclusion of intervention related content.

Content	MCP	CCST	Definition
Treatment Goal	X	X	Exploring the meaning of life after a cancer diagnosis by sharing thoughts and feelings between the cancer patient and their caregivers and facilitating a greater understanding of possible sources of meaning before and after the diagnosis and making decisions or solving problems
Communication Skill: Speaker		X	Guidelines for sharing thoughts and feelings
Communication Skill: Listen		X	Guidelines for listening to others' thoughts and feelings
The will to Meaning	X		The need to find meaning in our existence is a basic primary motivating force shaping human behavior.
Freedom of will	X		We have the "freedom" to find meaning in our existence and to choose our attitude toward suffering.
Life has meaning	X		Frankl believed that life has meaning and never ceases to have meaning, or the potential for meaning, from the first moments of life up to the end.
Homework: Encountering Life's Limitations	X		Three question exercise regarding encountering life's limitations.
Identity	X		Our identity is significantly influenced by the people, roles, and other aspects of our life that give our lives meaning.
Experiential Sources of Meaning	X		Connecting w/life through love, relationships, beauty, nature, and humor.
Creative Sources of Meaning	X		Actively engaging in life via work, deeds, accomplishments/via courage, commitment, responsibility
Homework: Share Your Legacy~Tell Your Story and Legacy Project	X		Tell your story to loved ones in your life in any manner that is comfortable to you.
Homework: Connecting with Life	X		List three ways in which you "connect with life" and feel most alive through the experiential sources of love, humor, and beauty.
Four sessions		X	Content presented in four sessions
Family integration		X	The integration of family into therapy

3. Analysis

Descriptive statistics were conducted using IBM SPSS Statistics 21 to examine the demographic and acceptance questionnaires. The semi-structured interview analyses, integration, and interpretation were completed in Spanish. A coding dictionary was developed and defined a priori, following standard deductive analysis procedures [5,6,16,17], which included developing a structured coding matrix with categories, codes, and definitions [5,6,16,17]. The qualitative codes used for the interviews included high, moderate, low, and neutral acceptance. Acceptance was noted as high when the patient or caregiver clearly stated that he or she liked the definition/question/exercise; as moderate when the patient or caregiver reported that he or she moderately liked the content or they liked it but felt that other patients or caregivers might not; and low when the patient or caregiver reported not liking the content. When the level of acceptance could not be established, it was coded as neutral.

Using the report and query functions of ATLAS.ti, the qualitative analysts (CP, LR, and KS) independently coded the transcripts and discussed divergence and convergence points [5,6,16,17]. The qualitative coders then coded the remaining transcriptions using the coding dictionary, and meetings were held to reach a consensus about the applied codes. Through consensus meetings, divergence, and convergence, points were discussed in the group until consensus was met. There were no significant differences between the coders, and if there was a difference (two to one), a consensus was reached after discussion. Reliability was conducted through team-based consensus building. The team's previous publications include more details about the methodology [15–18]. All investigators had expertise in qualitative analysis, and the last author moderated these discussions [15–18].

4. Results

Demographic survey. Fourteen patient–caregiver dyads completed the demographic and acceptance questionnaire. The patients' mean age was 59 years (SD = 11, range = 40–76), 57% were female, and 100% were Latinx. Patients' diagnoses included stage III cancer (n = 3) and stage IV cancer (n = 10). The caregivers' mean age was 52 years (SD = 13, range = 25–79), 57% were female, and 100% were Latinx. Among the caregivers, 9 were spouses or husbands (64.2%), 2 sisters (14.2%), 1 daughter (7.2%), 1 grandson (7.2%), and 1 friend (7.2%).

Acceptance questionnaires. Twelve patients (85.7%) and eleven caregivers (78.6%) reported high acceptance of the treatment goal. The acceptance data are summarized, and the separate voices of patients and caregivers are included in Table 2.

Table 2. Descriptive statistics for the acceptance questionnaire.

Content	N Patients	% Patients	N Caregivers	% Caregivers
Treatment Goal	12	85.7%	11	78.6%
Communication Skill: Speaker	13	92.9%	14	100%
Communication Skill: Listen	12	85.%	12	85.7%
The Will to Meaning	14	100%	11	78.6%
Identity	12	85.7%	13	92.9%
Experiential Sources of Meaning	12	85.7%	13	92.9%
Homework: Share Your Legacy~Tell Your Story and Legacy Project	12	85.7%	14	100%
Homework: Connecting with Life	14	100%	13	92.9%
Family integration	12	85.7%	12	85.7%

4.1. Treatment Goal

The goal of the intervention consists of exploring the meaning of life after a cancer diagnosis by sharing thoughts and feelings between cancer patients and their caregivers, facilitating a greater understanding of possible sources of meaning before and after the diagnosis, and making decisions or solving problems. On the acceptance questionnaire, patients (n = 12) and caregivers (n = 11) reported high acceptance of the intervention (see Table 2). In the qualitative interview, thirteen participants' responses were categorized with high acceptance of the treatment goal (see Table 3). See also the illustrative quotations in Table 4.

Table 3. High, moderate, low, and neutral acceptance of the intervention.

Categories	Themes	Response
High acceptance of intervention content	Treatment Goal	12
	Communication Skill: Speaker	14
	Communication Skill: Listen	13
	The will to meaning	10
	Life has a meaning	10
	Freedom of will	11
	Homework: Encountering Life's Limitations	10
	Identity	12
	Experiential	12
	Creative sources of meaning	13
	Homework: Share Your Legacy~Tell Your Story and Legacy Project	10
	Homework: Connecting with life	13
	4 sessions	10
Moderate acceptance of of intervention content	Homework: Encountering life's limitations	2
	Identity	1
	Experiential	1
	Creative sources of Meaning	1
	Homework: Share Your Legacy~Tell Your Story and Legacy Project	2
Low acceptance of intervention content	Treatment Goal	2
	The will to Meaning	1
	Life has meaning	1
	Freedom of will	1
	Homework: Encountering Life's Limitations	1
	Experiential	1
	Homework: Share Your Legacy~Tell Your Story and Legacy Project	2
	4 sessions	2
Neutral	Communication Skill: Listen	1
	The will to Meaning	1
	Life has meaning	3
	Freedom of will	2
	Communication Skill: Listen	1
	Homework: Encountering Life's Limitations	1
	Identity	1
	Homework: Connecting with Life	1
	4 sessions	2

Table 4. Caregivers–Patients Support to Latinx coping advanced-cancer (CASA) illustrative quotations for the high acceptance themes.

Themes	Illustrative Quotations for High Acceptance
Treatment Goal	Regarding the intervention's treatment goal, caregiver #3 expressed: "I think, I think it is really, really good. Since, well, how do you say it? Because it helps."
Communication Skill: Speaker	Regarding communication skills as a speaker sharing their thoughts and emotions, caregiver #5 expressed: "Well, how can I say it? Yes, they are important. They are good because one must learn to communicate, learn to express what one feels."

Table 4. *Cont.*

Themes	Illustrative Quotations for High Acceptance
Communication Skill: Listen	Regarding communication skills as a listener when the speaker is communicating, caregiver #12 expressed: "Yes, it seems fine to me. It is a way to follow some steps that can lead you to not interrupt that person who is perhaps expressing themselves at that moment, saying how they feel and letting you go through these steps. Then you can say: 'let me hold on and let the person finish, even if I have any questions.' Because, of course, they can be speaking, the person may be speaking. And if I interrupted them, interrupted them for a moment, I stopped the thought process they were having."
The will to meaning, life has meaning and freedom of will	Regarding the need to find meaning in their life, patient #13 expressed: "I liked it . . . I liked two, the will to meaning (desire for meaning) and freedom of will (free will) because I believe that there are decisions or attitudes towards life, in the face of this situation that happened to me, as well as other people. And I think that you must face it, as you say, on the battlefield where you must fight every day." Regarding Frankl's approach to life and meaning, patient #14 expressed: "That life has a meaning was very important, now that we went back.' People say, 'one comes here just to suffer,', but it always has meaning." Regarding the freedom to find meaning in our lives and chosen attitudes toward suffering, caregiver #12 expressed: "That sounds interesting because, if you are telling me, to put a situation here, a family member dies, my father died, or someone . . . Well, I have freedom of will (free will) to choose how I feel in that situation. That's what I'm understanding from what you are telling me. I find that reflection curious, that this person had, that any person, every person, has freedom of will (free will) to choose how they are going to feel, how they should face that situation. Regardless as I understand it, any person has that right or has the freedom of will (free will), but it's not easy and not everyone can achieve it."
Identity	Regarding identity, its influences, and its relationship to the meaning of life, patient #2 expressed: "I like it, because obviously one's feelings on how one is, how one was and how one is and was after the . . . (referring to diagnosis)."
Experiential and creative sources of Meaning	Regarding the ways a person experiences and connects with life through love, beauty, nature, humor, or relationships, patient #14 expressed: "Yes, because not everyone has the same problem or, no matter what the problem is, not everyone can play the same way and anything you can contribute to help someone or, at least, visualize that you have . . . but a problem and how you can resolve it and how they can endure everything. I bet that it is welcomed." Regarding how a person actively engages in life through work, deeds, and accomplishments, caregiver #5 expressed: "Very good, they are interesting."
Homework: Share Your Legacy~Tell Your Story and Legacy Project	Regarding an assignment where the participant creates a project that integrates meaning, identity, and creativity to generate a sense of meaning in light of their life and diagnosis, caregiver #12 expressed: "It's a good thing and in the end, the person thinks about this and has the desire to think: 'Before I leave, I want to leave with a grand finale (gold medal). I want to travel, if I want to travel; I want to eat all the ice cream in the ice cream shop.' Whatever it may be. 'Let's do this that I have never done before and always wanted, let's do it.'"
Homework: Connecting with Life	Regarding an assignment where the participant lists how they connect with life through love, beauty, and humor, patient #14 expressed: "All of them lead you to be what you are as a human being. With one you are more open, and others are less open, but all of them lead us there."

Table 4. Cont.

Themes	Illustrative Quotations for High Acceptance
Family integration	Regarding the integration of a family member into the intervention, caregiver #4 and patient #10 expressed: "As long as the person is in agreement, yes." Caregiver # 4 "Yes, because sometimes it is important to include another person. Yes." Patient #10
Four sessions	Regarding the acceptance of an intervention with four sessions, patient #1 expressed: There would be four, because there is time to develop the topics.

4.2. Communication Skills Training

The communication skills training includes components to assist couples in communicating effectively (e.g., how to speak and listen), decreasing the avoidance of critical cancer-related issues, and supporting each other. On the acceptance questionnaire, patients (n = 13) and caregivers (n = 14) reported high acceptance of the communication skills training speaker technique (see Table 2). Moreover, patients (n = 12) and caregivers (n = 12) reported high acceptance of the listening technique in the communication skills training (see Table 2). Thirteen participants' responses were categorized as high acceptance regarding how to listen to instructions. In the qualitative interview, all 14 participants' responses were categorized as high acceptance of the how-to-speak instructions (Table 3).

4.3. Meaning Content

On the acceptance questionnaire (see Table 2), patients (n = 14) and caregivers (n = 11) reported high acceptance of the will to meaning content. The meaning content is based on the principles of Viktor Frankl's work and his concepts of logotherapy by enhancing a sense of meaning, peace, and purpose as they approach the end of life. Patients (n = 12) and caregivers (n = 13) reported high acceptance of the identity content and experiential sources of meaning content. Patients (n = 12) and caregivers (n = 14) also reported high acceptance of the Homework: Share Your Legacy task, and patients (n = 14) and caregivers (n = 13) also reported high acceptance of the Homework: Connecting with Life task (see Table 2).

In the semi-structured interviews (see Table 3), the content identity and experiential sources of meaning were categorized as high acceptance, with 12 participants responding (see Table 3). The sources' meaning content was categorized as high acceptance for 13 participants. The content related to freedom of will was categorized as high acceptance, with 11 responses. The content related to will meaning and life has meaning was categorized as high acceptance, with 10 responses. Regarding the meaning content of homework, connecting with life, the response of 13 participants was categorized as high acceptance. Ten responses were categorized as high acceptance regarding the Encountering Life's Limitations and Legacy Project homework. When asked about the will to include the Legacy Project homework, 12 participants' responses were categorized as high acceptance. Regarding the Connecting with Life homework, 11 participants' responses were categorized as high acceptance.

4.4. Intervention Format

On the acceptance questionnaire, patients (n = 12) and caregivers (n = 12) reported high acceptance when asked about family integration into the therapy sessions (see Table 2). When asked about session intervention length, in the semi-structured interviews, 10 participants' responses were categorized as high acceptance, two as low acceptance, and two as neutral (Table 3).

4.5. Integration of the Findings to Protocol

The text was independently reviewed, followed by consensus meetings to discuss every intervention session, provide feedback, and discuss further modifications until a consensus was reached. The most accepted content of Caregivers-Patients Support to Latinx coping advanced-cancer (CASA) was included [17]. The cultural expert (NTB) and collaborators (CP, LR, and KS) conducted the integration of the qualitative findings to develop the CASA fixed in Table 5. The most commonly endorsed content of the CASA intervention was Communication Skills: Speaker, followed by Communication Skill: Listen, Creative Sources of Meaning, and Homework: Connecting with Life. The treatment goal, the content related to identity, and the experiential sources of meaning were also accepted, as were freedom of will, the will to meaning, life has meaning, Encountering Life's Limitations, and the Legacy project.

Table 5. CASA components that were culturally and linguistically adapted and integrated after the interviews and feedback. The X indicate the inclusion of intervention related content and the cultural adaptation.

Content	Included	Culturally Adapted	Adaptation
Treatment Goal	X	X	We include an introduction section to discuss the treatment goal and learn about cancer experience.
Communication Skill: Speaker	X	X	We include the CCST guidelines for sharing thoughts and feelings in session one
Communication Skill: Listen	X	X	We include the CCST guidelines for listening to others' thoughts and feelings in session one
The will to Meaning	X	X	We include meaning-centered content in session three.
Identity	X	X	We include identity content in session two.
Experiential Sources of Meaning	X	X	We include experiential sources of meaning content in session three.
Homework: Share Your Legacy~Tell Your Story and Legacy Project	X	X	We include the Legacy project on session two homework
Homework: Connecting with Life	X		We include the Legacy project on session three homework
4 sessions		X	Content change to be presented in 4 sessions
Family integration	X	X	We integrate family related content to the intervention

Dr. Rosario Costas Muñiz, the treatment and cultural expert, reviewed the text to ensure the adaptation considers the dimensions of the ecological validity model, a framework used to create culturally sensitive interventions for Hispanics [18]. Fidelity to CASA's concepts, goals, and a theoretical model was preserved during the adaptation process to ensure language, metaphor, strategy, cultural context, and value acceptance. See Table 5 to see the intervention protocol's content and adaptation.

5. Discussion

This study aimed to obtain patient-caregiver dyads' initial evaluation of the Caregivers-Patients Support to Latinx coping advanced-cancer (CASA) protocol, specifically tailored to address spirituality and communication among Latinx patients. Included in this brief report were results from the interviews conducted with patients and caregivers to help adjust and refine the protocol. Based on the findings of the acceptance questionnaire and the semi-structured interviews, the study team refined the intervention content and format.

Latinx patients and caregivers described the communication skills content as highly acceptable and relevant to coping with patient and caregiver needs. The most endorsed content of the CASA intervention was Communication Skills: Speaker, followed by Communication Skill: Listen. These findings are consistent with the literature [6,7] suggesting the acceptance of incorporating communication skills training in patients-caregivers coping with cancer. The team only includes the most acceptable content for the adaptation of CASA. These include incorporating the content endorsed by the caregivers and patients through the semi-structured interview related to Creative Sources of Meaning, identity, and experiential Sources of Meaning. Participants also reported high acceptance of freedom of will, followed by the Will to Meaning, Life has a Meaning and Homework Encountering life limitations and Legacy project. This acceptable content was similar to the team's previous research in adapting individual meaning-centered psychotherapy (IMCP) for Latinxs [6]. We also integrate the adapted protocol's most accepted intervention homework by patients and caregivers: the Legacy project and Connecting with Life.

Concerning the format of CASA, many participants preferred sessions accompanied by caregivers; however, some patient–caregiver pairs reported the barrier of attending simultaneously. Thus, the intervention length was refined based on the findings of the semi-structured interview and recommendations of the cultural expert. As suggested in the findings from the acceptance survey, the format of the CASA intervention will need to match the needs and resources of patients and caregivers (e.g., videoconferences, telephone intervention, or home visits). As evidenced by the present study, most participants reported high acceptance of incorporating caregivers into the intervention and high acceptance of the intervention length.

6. Conclusions

In conclusion, patient–caregiver dyads found CASA's communication and meaning content acceptable, as evidenced in the acceptance survey and semi-structured interviews. Additionally, caregivers and patients expressed the acceptance of participating in this intervention together. The results make the CASA adaptation an essential step towards refinement and piloting with Latinx families coping with advanced cancer. Furthermore, including communication skills and meaning-centered content will assist Latinx patients and caregivers with their palliative and end-of-life decision-making.

Implementing CASA in different communities is feasible because of this study's variety of patients and types of cancers. However, cultural differences should be considered. This study may contribute to the development of cultural adaptations by proving sensitive ways to conduct interventions. Given the heterogeneity of Latinx culture, it will provide a practical way to facilitate the way interventions are conducted with Latinx patients. This line of research's future direction should include the adapted intervention's pilot test.

7. Limitation

Consenting with patients and caregivers and collecting data remotely were challenging and time-consuming. An additional limitation was that the team did not include a pilot test of the intervention. We also did not have sexual orientation and sexual identity in the demographic data. By not collecting this critical information, we could not divide the responses by gender or sexual identity or consider the gender of the interviewer for the results of this study. For future studies, we should consider the participants' sexual orientation and sexual identity to report findings. Nonetheless, these preliminary findings suggest that a patient–caregiver intervention is acceptable and may be a promising approach to managing spirituality and communication in patients and caregivers coping with advanced cancer.

Author Contributions: Conceptualization, N.T.-B., L.P., E.M.C.-F., M.S., W.B. and R.C.-M.; methodology, N.T.-B. and R.C.-M.; software, L.R., C.P.-V., K.S. and N.T; validation, N.T.-B., R.C.-M. and E.M.C.-F.; formal analysis, L.R., C.P.-V., Y.T.-M. and K.S.; investigation, N.T.-B.; resources, N.T.-B. and E.M.C.-F.; data curation, L.R., C.P.-V., K.S. and N.T.-B.; writing—original draft preparation; writing N.T.-B.—review and editing, N.T.-B. and R.C.-M.; visualization, N.T.-B.; supervision, L.P., E.M.C.-F., M.S., W.B. and R.C.-M.; project administration, N.T.-B.; funding acquisition, N.T.-B. All authors have read and agreed to the published version of the manuscript.

Funding: This research was funded by the National Institute of Minority Health and Health Disparities (5G12MD007579, 5R25MD007607, R21MD013674, and 5U54MS007579-35); National Cancer Institute National Cancer Institute (2U54CA163071 and 2U54CA163068), R21CA180831-02 (Cultural Adaptation of Meaning-Centered Psychotherapy for Latinos), 1R25CA190169-01A1 (Meaning-Centered Psychotherapy Training for Cancer Care Providers), 5K08CA234397 (Adaptation and Pilot Feasibility of a Psychotherapy Intervention for Latino with Advanced Cancer) and the Memorial Sloan Kettering Cancer Center grant (P30CA008748). Supported in part by 133798-PF-19-120-01-CPPB from the American Cancer Society.

Institutional Review Board Statement: This project was revised and approved by the Ponce Health Sciences University–Ponce Research Institute Review Board (IRB). It complies with the United States 45 Code of Federal Regulations part 46 (45 CFR 46) related to the Common Rule and human subject regulation.

Informed Consent Statement: Informed consent was obtained from all subjects involved in the study.

Data Availability Statement: Not applicable.

Conflicts of Interest: The authors declare no conflict of interest.

References

1. Miller, K.D.; Ortiz, A.P.; Pinheiro, P.S.; Bandi, P.; Minihan, A.; Fuchs, H.E.; Martinez Tyson, D.; Tortolero-Luna, G.; Fedewa, S.A.; Jemal, A.M. Cancer statistics for the US Hispanic/Latino population, 2021. *CA Cancer J. Clin.* **2021**, *71*, 466–487. [CrossRef]
2. AARP and National Alliance for Caregiving. *Caregiving in the United States 2020*; AARP: Washington, DC, USA, 2020. [CrossRef]
3. Samuel, C.A.; Mbah, O.M.; Elkins, W.; Pinheiro, L.C.; Szymeczek, M.A.; Padilla, N.; Walker, J.S.; Corbie-Smith, G. Calidad de Vida: A systematic review of quality of life in Latino cancer survivors in the USA. *Qual. Life Res.* **2020**, *29*, 2615–2630. [CrossRef] [PubMed]
4. Hunter-Hernández, M.; Costas-Muñíz, R.; Gany, F. Missed opportunity: Spirituality as a bridge to resilience in Latinos with cancer. *J. Relig. Health* **2015**, *54*, 2367–2375. [CrossRef] [PubMed]
5. Costas-Muñíz, R.; Garduño-Ortega, O.; Torres-Blasco, N.; Castro-Figueroa, E.; Gany, F. "Maintaining hope:" challenges in counseling latino patients with advanced cancer. *J. Psychosoc. Oncol. Res. Pract.* **2020**, *2*, e028. [CrossRef] [PubMed]
6. Costas-Muñíz, R.; Torres-Blasco, N.; Castro-Figueroa, E.M.; González, C.J.; Breitbart, W.; Gany, F. Meaning-centered psychotherapy for Latino patients with advanced cancer: Cultural adaptation process. *J. Palliat. Med.* **2020**, *23*, 489–497. [CrossRef] [PubMed]
7. Torres-Blasco, N.; Castro, E.; Crespo-Martín, I.; Gonzalez, K.; Ramirez, E.P.; Garduño, O.; Costas-Muñíz, R. Comprehension and acceptance of the Meaning-Centered Psychotherapy with a Puerto Rican patient diagnosed with advanced cancer: A case study. *Palliat. Supportive Care* **2020**, *18*, 103–109. [CrossRef] [PubMed]
8. Ting, A.; Lucette, A.; Carver, C.S.; Cannady, R.S.; Kim, Y. Preloss spirituality predicts postloss distress of bereaved cancer caregivers. *Ann. Behav. Med.* **2019**, *53*, 150–157. [CrossRef] [PubMed]
9. Hall, G.C.N.; Ibaraki, A.Y.; Huang, E.R.; Marti, C.N.; Stice, E. A meta-analysis of cultural adaptations of psychological interventions. *Behav. Ther.* **2016**, *47*, 993–1014. [CrossRef] [PubMed]
10. Griner, D.; Smith, T.B. Culturally adapted mental health intervention: A meta-analytic review. *Psychother. Theory Res. Pract. Train.* **2006**, *43*, 531. [CrossRef] [PubMed]
11. Benish, S.G.; Quintana, S.; Wampold, B.E. Culturally adapted psychotherapy and the legitimacy of myth: A direct-comparison meta-analysis. *J. Couns. Psychol.* **2011**, *58*, 279. [CrossRef] [PubMed]
12. Smith, T.B.; Rodríguez, M.D.; Bernal, G. Culture. *J. Clin. Psychol.* **2011**, *67*, 166–175. [CrossRef] [PubMed]
13. Kreling, B.; Selsky, C.; Perret-Gentil, M.; Huerta, E.E.; Mandelblatt, J.S. 'The worst thing about hospice is that they talk about death': Contrasting hospice decisions and experience among immigrant Central and South American Latinos with US-born White, non-Latino cancer caregivers. *Palliat. Med.* **2010**, *24*, 427–434. [CrossRef] [PubMed]

14. Hsieh, H.-F.; Shannon, S.E. Three approaches to qualitative content analysis. *Qual. Health Res.* **2005**, *15*, 1277–1288. [CrossRef] [PubMed]
15. Braun, V.; Clarke, V. Using thematic analysis in psychology. *Qual. Res. Psychol.* **2006**, *3*, 77–101. [CrossRef]
16. Torres-Blasco, N.; Castro-Figuero, E.; Garduño-Ortega, O.; Costas-Muñiz, R. Cultural Adaptation and Open Pilot of Meaning-Centered Psychotherapy for Puerto Rican Patients with Advanced Cancer. *Sci. J. Educ.* **2020**, *8*, 100. [CrossRef] [PubMed]
17. Torres-Blasco, N.; Muñiz, R.C.; Zamore, C.; Porter, L.; Claros, M.; Bernal, G.; Shen, M.J.; Breitbart, W.; Castro, E. Cultural adaptation of meaning-centered psychotherapy for latino families: A protocol. *BMJ Open* **2022**, *12*, e045487. [CrossRef] [PubMed]
18. Bernal, G.; Bonilla, J.; Bellido, C. Ecological validity and cultural sensitivity for outcome research: Issues for the cultural adaptation and development of psychosocial treatments with Hispanics. *J. Abnorm. Child Psychol.* **1995**, *23*, 67–82. [CrossRef] [PubMed]

MDPI
St. Alban-Anlage 66
4052 Basel
Switzerland
www.mdpi.com

Healthcare Editorial Office
E-mail: healthcare@mdpi.com
www.mdpi.com/journal/healthcare

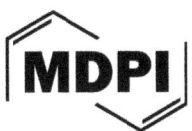

Disclaimer/Publisher's Note: The statements, opinions and data contained in all publications are solely those of the individual author(s) and contributor(s) and not of MDPI and/or the editor(s). MDPI and/or the editor(s) disclaim responsibility for any injury to people or property resulting from any ideas, methods, instructions or products referred to in the content.

www.ingramcontent.com/pod-product-compliance
Lightning Source LLC
LaVergne TN
LVHW070045120526
838202LV00101B/515